Jon,
Celebrate Ed
as a precious gift
Bobbi de Cordova-N

To my prayer partner Jon,
Prepare for
the best!

Tears
of
Joy

In Sickness and in Health
a Cancer Survivor
and Caregiver
Share Their Story

by Jerry Hanks and
Bobbi de Córdova-Hanks

Copyright © 2003, 2006 by
Jerry Hanks & Bobbi de Córdova-Hanks

Second Edition

All rights reserved. No part of this book shall be reproduced or transmitted in any form or by any means, electronic, mechanical, magnetic, photographic including photocopying, recording or by any information storage and retrieval system, without prior written permission of the publisher. No patent liability is assumed with respect to the use of the information contained herein. Although every precaution has been taken in the preparation of this book, the publisher and author assume no responsibility for errors or omissions. Neither is any liability assumed for damages resulting from the use of the information contained herein.

ISBN 0-7414-1444-9

Published by:

INFI∞ITY
PUBLISHING.COM

1094 New DeHaven Street, Suite 100
West Conshohocken, PA 19428-2713
Info@buybooksontheweb.com
www.buybooksontheweb.com
Toll-free (877) BUY BOOK
Local Phone (610) 941-9999
Fax (610) 941-9959

Printed in the United States of America

Printed on Recycled Paper

Published March 2007

Contents

Dedication i
Acknowledgments iii
Foreword v
Introduction vii

1. The Journey Begins 1
2. The Final Goodbye 4
3. Paying the Price of Ignorance 7
4. Bubba . . .and the Year After 10
5. Becoming an Amazon Warrior Woman 15
6. Bobbi and Bernard's 19
7. Does Anybody Have Two Nipples for a Dime? ... 23
8. From Dinner to Detection 31
9. Bosom Buddies on the Road 35
10. The Little Old Lady in Vancouver 41
11. Survivor -- From the Moment of Diagnosis 44
12. How to Be a Good Caregiver 49
13. The Faces of Courage 54
14. Getting Mad and Shedding Tears 57
15. The Second Time Around 62
16. Fighting the Good Fight 67
17. "Beam Me Up, Scotty" 71
18. Breast Cancer: Past, Present and Future 77

19. "Get a Life." I'd Love One, Thank You! 81
20. "The Good News of Survival" 85
21. "Heroes Are Everywhere" 91
22. "On the Road for Life" 98
23. The Next Bend in the Road 102
24. Prepare for the Best 106

Dedication

This book is dedicated to all breast cancer survivors everywhere who, like the butterfly, are symbols of hope and inspiration. . .

And to their caregivers who toil tirelessly to see that their hope never dims, inspired by the courage of those they care for.

And to the memory of Bobbi's Mother Florence who taught all who knew her about the true meaning of survival.

Acknowledgments

This book would double in size if we were to acknowledge everyone who has helped us along the way or spurred us on with words of encouragement.

Certainly the contributions of Jennifer Holland in designing the cover are worthy of special note. This is also true for the contributions of Pat McSweeney, our "ghost editor" supreme; Pat Klaus, for her untiring creative efforts; Mike Rosenberg, our long-suffering and incredibly talented computer genius, and Mike Dowling, our agent for speaking engagements and an author himself, who urged us forward when the trail got murky.

To all of them, and to all whose names are mentioned in the pages of this book, we owe our heartfelt gratitude.

Bobbi and Jerry
Jacksonville, Florida
December 2006

Foreword

The Butterfly ... The Miracle

What is lovelier than the sight of a summery butterfly, dancing in flight as it flutters its beautiful velvety wings? What is miraculous is that it came forth in all its wonder, from its humbler state as a lovely, earthbound caterpillar. From cocoon-encased larva, to slow traveling caterpillar, to the beauteous creature in flight, the metamorphosis is a seeming miracle.

Similarly, a woman diagnosed with breast cancer can undergo a miraculous metamorphosis. First there is the period of darkness when we wrap ourselves in the cocoon of our personal struggle. Then we emerge reluctantly into the light of day to hesitantly embrace the truth of our unwelcome but unalterable situation. Then, at last, we arise into the potential of our newly appreciated freedom, freer of spirit, more graceful of mind, and more beautiful than before.

When facing despair, think of the butterfly as a symbol of hope and inspiration.

Author Unknown

Introduction

When we set out to write this book, one of the biggest challenges we faced was what to call it. We pretty much knew what we wanted to say and how we wanted to say it. But coming up with a title was a far different matter.

Bobbi's choice for the title was, "Does Anybody Have Two Nipples for a Dime? Breast Cancer...the Story of Change." Jerry didn't fail to see the humor but he feared the title would make the book sound overly frivolous.

Twenty-four chapters later we agreed on "Tears of Joy" as an acceptable compromise. Tears because there is no cancer journey without them. Joy because few people ever think about the other side of cancer -- the triumphs; the laughs; the friends you never knew you had and the new ones you meet along the way, and that strange sense of accomplishment that comes from knowing you have faced the worst and made the best of it.

And that's what this book is all about. Seven simple words. "Facing the worst" and "preparing for the best."

Some parts of the book may make you cry. Some may make you smile -- or even laugh out loud. A few parts are guaranteed to make you mad. And some, we hope, will make you cheer.

But that's what the cancer journey is all about. It's all right here and it's all true to the best of our memories and those of our friends.

We hope you will enjoy what we have to say and be inspired to make the most of your experience with cancer.

Jerry Hanks and Bobbi de Córdova-Hanks

1

Bobbi's Story...

The Journey Begins

When I first said the words "cancer survivor" in May 1986, I never realized they would become two of the most important words in my life.

I remember the experience vividly. I was walking through the corridor of Jacksonville International Airport on the way to meet my mother and sister who were coming from out of town to be with me for my mastectomy surgery. Two days before I had had a lumpectomy to remove a very large tumor, leaving me with an enormous amount of staples across my chest. As I walked through security . . . the alarm sounded.

As I searched through my pockets to see if my keys were there, I suddenly realized it was the staples that had set the alarm off. I called one of the female security officers to one side and told her, "I'm a cancer survivor and I just had surgery that left staples across my chest. Tomorrow I'm having my breast removed and I'm here to meet my family, who are coming to be with me." She immediately said not to worry, gently patted me down, walked me alongside the official security entrance and wished me Godspeed.

On the way down that very long corridor I thought how easily I had said "cancer survivor." I never said "victim." I said survivor, and for the first time since my diagnosis several days before, I saw a light at the end of the tunnel. I made a conscious choice at that very moment to focus on life and not on the disease.

When my mother and sister and I walked past security, I gave them the thumbs-up sign and they all stood there and applauded, saying they would keep me in their prayers. How could I possibly lose the battle when even total strangers were praying for me?

It was a beautiful spring day in May when my husband Jerry, my mother and I sat in the doctor's office and heard the doctor say, "It doesn't look good. It's malignant." I remember turning and looking over my shoulder to find the person he was talking about. I knew it couldn't be me. There was no history of breast cancer in my family and I was healthy as a horse. I had played three hours of tennis singles in scorching 93-degree temperature over the preceding weekend.

After realizing he was talking about me, my first thought was -- why doesn't he come out and say "cancer?" He used words like tumor, growth, malignancy, it looks serious, and many other words but never actually said you have cancer. That was my first glimpse of the fact that back in 1986, there seemed to be a stigma attached to having cancer and often people diagnosed with the disease felt the need to hide it.

After learning that I had advanced breast cancer that had spread to my lymph nodes and that I would undergo chemotherapy, I proceeded to educate myself on what was in store for me. I found that oncologists (a new word in my vocabulary at that time) were like grim reapers. They felt obliged to tell you all the terrible statistics and all the bad things that could happen to you.

Always an activist around one cause or another, my first thought was to prove their statistics wrong. Statistics are written about dead people and here I was, very much alive and kicking. I wondered at the time how any mortal could possibly know when I was going to leave the planet. After all, my doctor put his pants on the same way my husband did, one leg at a time, so who was he to play God?

Little did I know that that fateful day was the beginning of my cancer journey. A journey fraught with challenges and changes, both physical and spiritual. A journey that would continue to evolve with change after change, including an unexpected diagnosis of another primary cancer in December of 1999.

2

Jerry's Story...

The Final Goodbye

I really didn't know Gifford Grange very well. Our firm had helped him win election to Jacksonville's City Council but I really knew Gifford more as a client than as a personal friend.

So I was surprised to hear his voice on the line when the phone in my office rang, late on that cold, gray February afternoon.

"Jerry," he said, very cautiously and deliberately, "I just wanted to call and tell you how sorry I was to hear about Sally. She was a wonderful, wonderful woman."

I thanked him and we talked for a minute or two and then he said, " Do you mind if I ask you a personal question? What are you doing in your office at a time like this?"

I told him I wasn't quite sure. "I just stopped by," I said. "I'm on my way to the airport to pick up my father who's flying in for the service tomorrow morning."

"Who's going with you?" Gifford asked.

"No one," I answered. "I'm going alone."

"Jerry," Gifford said, his voice suddenly very commanding, "you can't do that. You wait. I'll be right there."

Fifteen minutes later Gifford was in my office in the Gulf Life Building and he drove me to the airport and waited with me. It's good that he did. Dad's plane from Arkansas was more than five and one-half hours late and as I've thought about it over the years, there was no way I would have ever made it all by myself.

Discovering friends you never knew you had, like Gifford Grange, is one of the surprising joys of being a cancer caregiver. But that thought was far from my mind when Dad and I finally arrived at the house in the early hours of Tuesday morning. Before the clock on the mantle would strike 12, Sally would be laid to rest.

I had asked John Riley, the rector at All Saints Episcopal Church, if we could have music at the service and if the organist could play a hymn that was not in the Episcopal hymnal. I've never forgotten his response. He said, "Jerry, we will do whatever you want for Sally. Just tell me so we can find the music and the words and hand them out to everyone."

The church was filled with those whose lives Sally had touched in the 44 years that God had given her. As soon as Father Riley pronounced the final commendation, the organist launched into the opening chords of *The Battle Hymn of the Republic*. I wanted everyone to hear us in the farthest reaches of Jacksonville just as I wanted them to hear us in Heaven. Because I wanted the world to feel the triumph of the moment and the joy that Sally stood for.

Then we went to the cemetery and said goodbye.

For many years after that, people would tell me it was the greatest funeral they had ever attended. That may sound strange, but that's what I wanted. Because Sally was a winner. And nothing, not even cancer, was ever going to change that simple fact. Not in my mind. Or Sally's. Or anyone else's.

Late that afternoon, after everyone had left, Dad and I sat alone in the living room. The clouds from the morning and the day before had gone away and sunlight streamed in through the windows, casting lengthening shadows upon the floor.

We talked very quietly about a lot of things, none of them very important. At length, during a pause in the conversation, Dad said, "You know I'll stay here as long as you need me. But the day is going to come when you'll need to get on with living. Sally is gone. Her suffering is over. But you must go on. People will understand your loss and your sorrow. But someday you'll need to put the mourning behind you and get on with the business of living."

I nodded in silence. John Riley had told me the same thing, in almost the same words, a few days earlier when we had finished planning Sally's service.

So early the next afternoon, I took Dad to the airport and put him on a plane back to Arkansas.

Then I went home and Bubba and I started life all over.

3

Bobbi's Story . . .

Paying the Price of Ignorance

Deep down inside, I knew something was very wrong with me. The trouble was, I couldn't seem to convince any of my doctors that that was the case, despite the fact that it was my body and I knew it very well. Obviously much better than they did.

So I went on with my life. And what a glorious life it was at that point. I had finally found my soulmate, I had the dream job of a lifetime as the editor of an international music magazine after retiring from 25 years as a professional bass player traveling around the world, and I was getting used to my new marriage and my new hometown.

But underneath the happiness, a kernel of dread was building. My emotions began to roller coaster and my fatigue became almost unbearable. I went to my gynecologist faithfully every six months because of my fibrocystic breasts, and each time I saw him I told him of my worry about something being wrong. He called it early menopause, the beginning of the change of life, but never suggested a mammogram and never asked me if I examined my breasts.

I thought back to when I was in my early 30s and found a sizeable lump beneath the nipple of my breast. The doctor at that time thought the lump was suspicious. He removed the nipple and took out a walnut-size lump. I'll never forget his words to this day. He said, "You are one lucky lady. The lump is benign and more than that, women who have these kinds of lumps never have to worry about getting breast cancer." And I believed him!

If only I knew then what I know and preach now, that doctors rarely find the lumps because they don't know what's normal for our breasts. Only we know that. That's why monthly breast self-examination is so critical. How could I have been so ignorant? Having what I thought were no risk factors, and being told 20 years earlier that I'd never have a serious problem, breast cancer never entered my mind.

After playing three hours of singles tennis one blistering hot and humid Florida Sunday, I could no longer ignore my fatigue and lay down to rest. When I woke up a while later, I rolled over on my stomach and it suddenly felt like my breast had turned to stone. I called my husband Jerry and told him, "A foreign object has lodged itself in my breast. It feels like my breast is made of stone." Even then, breast cancer was the farthest thing from my mind. After feeling my breast, Jerry said he thought I should call the doctor and maybe even go to see him.

A few days later, I watched the doctor's face turn white as he examined my breast. He immediately set up an appointment with a surgeon.

After the surgeon examined my breast, he made an appointment for my first mammogram, at the age of 50. Shortly after that a surgical biopsy confirmed our worst fears. It was malignant and due to the huge size of the tumor, the surgeon felt a mastectomy was the only option I had. Still reeling from the diagnosis of advanced breast cancer, Jerry and I returned to the gynecologist, not to blame him but to ask about the surgeon's credentials. When he saw Jerry and I sitting in his office, he turned white once again and said, "I told you to have a mammogram."

After telling him that wasn't true, I told him not to worry, I wasn't there to blame him or sue him, I just wanted to be sure I was in good hands since my life was on the line. It was to be the last time that gynecologist ever set eyes on me.

Not only did my surgeon do a fine job, but he also was caring and compassionate as well. Over the years, as I became more and more involved in cancer survivorship, Dr. L. Alan Smith came to understand the importance of the mind/body connection that I believe so strongly in and of the difference that emotional support can make to newly diagnosed women. I like to think he also became a friend.

4

Jerry's Story...

Bubba...and the Year After

I never would have made it without Bubba. He was one of the greatest listeners I've ever known.
In the days and weeks and months that slowly passed after Sally was gone, Bubba and I would sit on the edge of the bed and talk, sometimes for an hour or more at a time.
We talked about the good times that Sally and I had together. And the times we played tennis and the places we visited and the friends we met. Sometimes we talked about Southeastern Executive Service, the business which I owned and Sally managed with such unbridled zeal. And we talked about Hanks-Livingston, Inc., the small public relations, advertising and professional writing firm which I also owned.
Bubba would peer intently into my eyes as I talked, never interrupting until I paused. Then he'd quietly offer what sounded like encouragement or understanding or whatever the mood called for. I tell people about Bubba today and when they find out he was a gray and white, long-haired cat, I always get this raised-eyebrow expression. But they didn't

know Bubba the way I did. In fact, I knew Bubba before he was even born.

For nearly a year after Sally and I were married, we lived in an apartment complex in Jacksonville. The lady across the hall, I think her name was Carol, had a tortoise-shell cat named Cloudy, who made our apartment her second home. Cloudy loved to probe all the darkest corners and when she wasn't doing that she'd curl up on my desk.

Over a period of time I noticed Cloudy seemed to be getting a little plump. I'd gently stroke her belly and sometimes I thought I could detect some tiny objects inside, but I wasn't sure so I didn't say anything to Sally or Carol.

One day I came home from work later than Sally and found her and Carol sobbing in the living room. Cloudy was missing. In a rare burst of genius I suspected what had happened. I went to the bedroom and approached the closet. A footstep away I heard a faint meow. And there on the floor, between a bowling ball and a suitcase, was Cloudy with three of the tiniest kittens I had ever seen. I could easily have held all of them in the palm of one hand.

One of them didn't even have any fur, just bare skin, some of it sort of a grayish color and some of it sort of a pinkish-white. In a few days the fur started growing and what had been gray skin became gray fur and what had been pinkish-white skin became white fur. (I've told that to a lot of people and I don't think anyone believes me.)

That was Bubba (who we discovered much later was really a girl) and for nearly 19 years he was one of the best friends I had. And also one of the smartest.

One of the things Bubba and I decided early on was that just because I was aching with heartbreak and loneliness was no reason to fall madly in love with the first member of the opposite sex who flashed me a sympathetic smile. We decided I should wait at least a year (or maybe forever) before even thinking about getting serious.

Another thing Bubba and I agreed on was that never, not ever, should I compare anyone with Sally. Sally was one of a kind and if I started measuring others against her, no one would ever have a chance. Including me.

A third thing Bubba and I came up was the two-part "Bubba Test." Every woman I met, or would meet as time went on, had to pass the Bubba Test. The first part was easy. The woman had to convince me that (a) she was a cat lover and (b) that she liked Bubba. I'm easy to fool so that wasn't much of a challenge.

The second part of the test was to convince Bubba of the same thing and for more than a year no one passed the test.

Bubba's decision was never long in coming. Always the perfect host, he'd allow himself to be petted or even picked up and held. But when Bubba made up his mind, he'd head for the sofa, jump up and promptly go to sleep. It was the ultimate tails-down. But Bubba did it so subtly that no one ever knew what was happening. Except for Bubba and me.

Still another thing Bubba and I decided was that I should bury myself in my work in the hope that this would help me keep my mind off everything that had happened during the previous 12 months. It proved to be good therapy.

Hanks-Livingston had often been neglected, especially in the final three or four months of Sally's illness, and now I needed to get things moving again. Our clients, without exception, during the whole period of time were totally supportive. I never heard a single grumble or complaint although I'm sure there were many unreturned phone calls and missed deadlines.

One of the clients was David Harrell, who was president of Jacksonville's City Council. Unlike Gifford Grange, who I knew mostly through political endeavors until the night he shared his life with me, I knew David more for the marketing and public relations work we did for his independent insurance agency. David was an avowed workaholic -- always in a rush and impatient with those who would mire him in needless details. Many people thought he was brusque and insensitive to their feelings.

One day I got a small white envelope in the mail and inside was a handwritten note:

Dear Jerry,

> *I just wanted you to know that my heart goes out to you and Sally. Please let me know if there is ever anything I can do or if there is ever anything you need -- and that includes money.*
>
> *Sincerely yours,*
> *David*

Several years later, David Harrell left Jacksonville and went to Atlanta. I don't know where he is today. I never took him up on his offer. But I still have his note as a reminder of his kindness and that of so many other people who came to my aid in those darkest of days.

Gradually, I began to put the pieces of Hanks-Livingston back together. Deciding what to do with Southeastern Executive Service was an entirely different matter.

Southeastern originally subleased six small offices from Gulf Life Insurance Company in the 24-story building in which I was located. Southeastern rented the offices to small businesses and provided them with phone answering, secretarial, photocopying and conference room services. I had always been fascinated by the concept and when the owner of the business mysteriously walked away from it, Rudy Wood, the building manager, suggested I take over the business for free (and he'd still keep getting the monthly rental on all of the space).

What Southeastern needed, I thought, was a good manager and that's where Sally fit in. I had known her for a few years and I was always impressed with her sales ability and her talent for working with people and getting things done.

We quickly agreed on terms and I casually asked her if she knew how to type, since the manager occasionally had to fill in for one of the other office workers. Sally didn't answer so I asked the question again.

"No," she snapped, "I don't know how to type. You asked me if I could start in two weeks and I said yes. In two weeks I'll know how to type."

I looked at her and she wasn't smiling. It was the first time I had ever seen the fire in her eyes. "You've got a deal," I said.

Two weeks later she took over Southeastern Executive Service. And she knew how to type. I still don't know how she did it.

In a little more than a year we had expanded Southeastern to 11 offices in the Gulf Life building and opened a similar operation with 11 leased spaces in the Independent Life building on the other side of the St. Johns River.

Then we started talking about franchising the concept in other cities in Florida and then expanding regionally and even nationally. We also planned to be among the first to computerize our secretarial services.

We knew we could do it because Sally could sell. One day when I was with her at Independent Life she sold a total stranger on our telephone answering service and the next office we had available -- all in the time it took the elevator to go from the 22nd floor to the main lobby.

Soon after that Sally became ill and all of the dreams drifted away.

Now that she was gone I had little enthusiasm for the business. One day, completely unannounced, a man showed up in the office and said he heard that I might be interested in selling Southeastern. Without asking my price, he offered exactly 10 times what our accountant thought the business was worth. The next day we closed the deal.

That night Bubba got an extra large serving of catnip. And we both felt better.

5

Bobbi's Story...

Becoming an Amazon Warrior Woman

What I remember most about hearing the diagnosis of cancer was the surreal feeling that came over me. Once I finally heard the doctor say *cancer,* my mind immediately shut down. Now I know that this is something that happens to almost everyone when first diagnosed. That's when a second set of ears becomes critical. Whatever I thought I heard the doctor say was almost opposite of what Jerry really heard the doctor say. It was almost like an out-of-body experience. It was eerie. It was as if I were looking down at a scene from a play. It was one I happened to be starring in, but I couldn't see it.

As I prepared for my mastectomy surgery, random thoughts kept running through my head. If they remove my breast, what will I put in my bra when I leave the hospital? What will the surgical scar be like? Will I be the same person I was before? So many questions and so few answers. In those days, very few doctors recognized the importance of the psychosocial effects of breast cancer.

The mind/body connection was just beginning to surface along with books written by Dr. Bernie Siegel and Dr. Carl Siminton. The two were among the first to recognize that you really can't separate the mind from the body. And what a blessing it was to be able to read and learn from these books that there *is* life after cancer. To me it was like someone suddenly threw me the lifeline I was looking for.

I became like a human sponge, soaking up every piece of information I could lay my hands on. There was no information superhighway in 1986. If there was, I must have taken the first off ramp and missed it completely. I didn't even know anyone who had had breast cancer. Well maybe I did, but they never admitted it. Cancer was still "The Big C" back then. Now I know that the "C" stands for courage, compassion and conquest. We become Amazon warrior women. We are ready to stand our ground against this faceless enemy.

The date was May 22, 1986. The week of Mother's Day. Ironically, it was the week I had decided to start playing bass again and was looking forward to working with a newly put together big band. Little did I know that I would never play bass professionally again. It wasn't the breast cancer that forced me to stop playing, I just wasn't the same person I was before. My priorities changed instantly. I said goodbye to those dreams at the same time I said goodbye to my breast. It was time for a change.

The surgery went smoothly but then my blood counts dropped dramatically. I needed a blood transfusion and was given three units of blood. It was just about the time hospitals started checking blood to make sure it was safe. AIDS loomed on the horizon. I think the blood transfusions scared my family more than the cancer did. How did they know the blood was safe? Who had checked it?

Just as the last drop of blood was going through the IV, a young nurse came in and said, "Oh icky, blood. None of us who work here would have a blood transfusion." I felt the hair stand up on the back on my neck as I quickly asked her about her concerns. Was it fear of AIDS?

She said, "Oh it's not just AIDS, it's hepatitis and all the other little buggers that scare us." I was too shocked to say anything as I felt the cold chill of fear creep through my beat-up body. What else might I be facing in the future?

During the week I spent in the hospital (yes, this was definitely before managed care), I found out that there were very few answers to my questions. I remember a lovely volunteer who tried to cheer me up when she visited. She was about 75, an avid golfer and a mother of 10 children. She had a tiny body with tiny breasts. She said I could be just like her and I thought "not likely." I found it depressing. Even though she meant well, I was 50, had never had children of my own, was an avid tennis player and had been left with one humongous breast that was slowly creeping toward my kneecap. If someone had told me I could commit suicide by shooting myself two inches below my left breast, I would have shot off my kneecap. I couldn't have been like her in the best of situations.

Spring was in the air the day I left the hospital. You could smell the blossoming flowers everywhere. Beautiful impatiens and begonias lined the streets along with blooming crepe myrtle trees. Jerry had gone out and traded our car in for a cherry red Chrysler New Yorker just to make my homecoming special. I sat on the passenger side clutching my purse to my chest, feeling like everyone was staring at me minus a breast. I couldn't wait to get inside the house.

My mother and sister were staying with us to help out. Friends were popping in and out of the house. The phone was ringing off the hook. Relatives from everywhere were coming out of every nook and cranny to pull together in a tight knit family circle. I remember my late Uncle Archie calling me to ask if I wanted him to tell me a story just like he did when I was a child and I was afraid because my father was dying from a heart disease. What a comfort family can be.

Shortly after that, the big crash came. Jerry was at work and my family had gone back to South Florida. I was alone in the house for the first time since my surgery and I said, "Oh my god! I have cancer and I could die." After giving way to the tears that had been pent up, I began to think about my life, about the positives and the negatives. I found the positives far outweighed the negatives. I was the same person I was before. I could sure save a lot of money on haircuts, thanks to chemo, and I wouldn't have to tweeze my eyebrows or shave my legs for a year. What a plus!

6

Jerry's Story . . .

Bobbi and Bernard's

A new client of Hanks-Livingston in the year after Sally's death was the National Association Insurance Managers. (No, I don't know what happened to the "of".) NAIM specialized in providing insurance for the hospitality industry, especially restaurants, motels and hotels. Its founder and president was Andy Cizek and he and I quickly developed a great relationship, at least partly, I always thought, because we both wore the same style of regimental stripe neckties.

Andy, it turned out, had a problem. *The Florida Restaurateur*, the official publication of the Florida Restaurant Association, refused to run NAIM's advertising because a personal rift had developed between Andy and the restaurant association's insurance consultant. Andy wanted to know if there was anything I could do to convince the magazine to accept his advertising.

The whole thing sounded a little strange but I told him I'd give it a try. I found out that the editor (and also advertising manager) of the magazine was someone with the name of Bobbi de Córdova and I called her to find out what was really going on.

Bobbi de Córdova proceeded to inform me that (a) her name was pronounced de Córdova, with the accent on the "Cor"; (b) that she had no idea what I was talking about, and (c) that she couldn't believe the magazine would ever refuse any legitimate advertising. She asked me to send her a proposed ad and promised she'd look into things.

A week later she called back to say that she had met with the executive director of the association and that the magazine was willing to accept NAIM's advertising but she wondered if some changes could be made in the ad to make the language more palatable to the association.

Andy Cizek at first was livid, but he finally agreed to a few minor revisions. That wasn't enough for the FRA but Bobbi won a few more concessions on her end and back and forth we went. Bobbi and I became like two opposing attorneys, polite and courteous but detached, she realizing who signed her paycheck while I clearly understood that Andy Cizek was a paying client.

Amazingly, we resolved all of the differences. Andy Cizek was happy; his ad would run in a magazine that reached all of the state's restaurateurs. And the FRA had a new full page, full color advertiser and supporter. The insurance consultant was forgotten. It was just before Christmas and in our final telephone conversation, I thanked Bobbi for being so patient, and especially for her professional objectivity, and we wished each other a happy holiday season. I wondered if we would ever talk again.

The holidays were lonely for Bubba and me. We decorated a Christmas tree which stood by itself in a corner of the living room. Everyone tried to be friendly and include me in their holiday plans. I appreciated their kindness but it just wasn't the same.

My children, J.R. and Lee, and their mother Linda, who was my wife long before Sally, were wonderful. So was my mother, who had moved to Jacksonville several years earlier. I would like to have seen Dad but my stepmother had become critically ill and Dad spent all of his time with her. So I was glad when the holidays were over and I had an excuse to bury myself in work again.

During the two-week break, Andy Cizek had decided we should do an entirely new ad for the *Florida Restaurateur*, and this precipitated a whole new round of talks with Bobbi de Córdova.

Our back and forth discussions started to become the highlight of my work and this time things went much more smoothly. When we finally came to closure, I was so relieved I said, "It's too bad you don't live in Jacksonville and I'd buy you a drink after work to celebrate."

"If I lived in Jacksonville, I just might accept," she shot back. Her answer caught me completely off guard and for the next several days I couldn't get it out of my mind. She actually sounded like she meant it!

I kept telling myself how stupid it was for me even to have asked the question. For all I knew, Bobbi de Córdova was happily married with a house full of children. But then I wondered. . .

A week later I found an excuse to call her again. She seemed pleased that I had called and after we had talked business for a minute I took a deep breath and said, "You sounded serious about having that drink after work."

I didn't know where the conversation would lead but I had decided to find out. "It's too bad it's 360 miles from Miami to Jacksonville," I said. "Maybe we should meet somewhere in between, like Orlando. That's only 200 miles for you and 140 for me, but we could also have dinner."

"Well," she said, "fair is fair."

"To be really fair," I said, pushing my luck all the way, "we should get together in Cocoa Beach. That would be about 180 miles for both of us. We could have dinner at Bernard's Surf. It's rated one of Florida's best restaurants and if you're not familiar with it, as editor of the *Florida Restaurateur* you should be. I used to be in the space program so I know the area. I could get you a room at the Holiday Inn and I'd stay with a friend in Cocoa Beach."

"Sounds great," Bobbi said with enthusiasm. "I've heard of Bernard's and might even consider it for a cover story. It all sounds like fun."

"How about a week from this Saturday?" I asked. "I'll make a reservation at Bernard's and get a room for you at the Holiday Inn. I'll pick you up at 7 o'clock."

When we hung up I was so excited I was actually trembling. That night I told Bubba what I had done. He listened in wide-eyed silence. Then he made a sort of quizzical sound and it struck me. Here I was, making a date to travel 180 miles, to have dinner at one of the finest restaurants in the state, with a woman -- and I didn't even know what she looked like.

7

Bobbi's Story...

Does Anybody Have Two Nipples for a Dime?

Life A. D. (after diagnosis) is filled with never ending change. You may wonder about the title of this chapter, "Does anybody have two nipples for a dime?" It's actually the punch line from a very old joke about a topless ticket taker and a reverend. I won't go into the details of the joke other than to say it seemed appropriate for a book about a cancer journey. A journey filled with twists and turns and change.

The analogy I like to use is that it's like crossing a river to the other side. You can never go back to the starting point again. Your friends can cross the river with you, but, unlike you, they can still journey between both sides of the river. That's what makes cancer so isolating. No one can say they know what you're going through unless they've walked in your shoes.

In the first days after diagnosis, I felt as though my life was a movie playing inside my head. I thought a lot about how Jerry and I met while I was editor of the *Florida*

Restaurateur magazine. I had taken a hiatus from dating after my divorce and here I was traveling almost 200 miles to meet someone I had only talked to over the telephone.

I remember asking my mother, who was then in her 70s, what she thought about this crazy idea of driving all the way to Cocoa Beach to have dinner with a man who could be two feet tall and four feet wide for all I knew. Much to my amazement, she actually encouraged me to go, saying, "If worst comes to worst, you have dinner and come home." She knew that I had enjoyed the conversations I had with Jerry while plotting how to make peace between our warring companies. I think she secretly felt I could use some excitement in my life at that point.

When the fateful day arrived, I got into my 1970 240Z Datsun and burned rubber on the way to Cocoa Beach. I was really brave about this until I checked into the Holiday Inn. Then I thought, "What have I done?" I didn't know what to expect, but for some reason I decided to go for broke. I wore an extremely low cut black jumpsuit (still having cleavage at that time) and four inch black silk heels. Little did I know that Jerry was wild about high heels. It was something he developed while working as the women's editor of the *Honolulu Star-Bulletin*. The only trouble was that I had just gone through one of those "I hate my hair" phases and had a military-type buzz cut with about two inches of hair left on my head.

When the appointed time came and he knocked at the door, I opened it up to see a wonderfully handsome man with a thick head of silver hair standing there. Wow! I had hit pay dirt! He was so dazzled by the high heels and cleavage that he never even noticed my hair.

After spending an incredible evening talking our way through dinner and some of Cocoa Beach's night spots, he took me back to the hotel and kissed me on the forehead. I didn't know whether to be glad or sad. Somehow I thought he'd be like all the other men I dated who took me out to dinner and then expected to dance the horizontal mambo.

I stood behind the closed door thinking about how much I had enjoyed the evening when there was a knock on the door. I looked out through the peep hole and there Jerry was. I opened the door expecting him to make a move when he said, "I don't know when I've had such a nice evening. Can I pick you up at 10 o'clock tomorrow for breakfast?"

When I left to return to Miami the next day, I wondered if I'd ever see him again. He said he'd be in touch and when several days passed with no phone call or letter (this was before e-mail), I thought he was just like the rest of the men in my life. Then I opened my mailbox and found a press release he had written about our meeting. The headline read, "NAIM Representative's Meeting with *Florida Restaurateur* Editor Exceeds Expectations." I knew at that moment that this would be a very special relationship.

My mother was right when she told me that every pot finds its cover. Not only did we both come from up north, and both had a love of words, but best of all we were both animal lovers. I remember Jerry asking me if I played tennis. I told him I did and then ran out to buy a racket, tennis skirt and top. Nothing was going to stand in the way of this relationship. Little did I know what fate had in store.

How could I put my husband Jerry through this again? Wasn't losing one wife to cancer enough? How could I voice my fears to someone who had experienced all that he went through with Sally? Would our lives ever be the same again? Would we live in fear forever? Would we play tennis again?

So much of our life revolved around playing tennis. We would only vacation in places that had tennis courts. And, believe me, we were very competitive. Jerry had devised a method that leveled the playing field for both of us, since he obviously was a stronger player. After I fine-tuned my game, I know he often thought that he probably should have rescinded the method.

A few weeks after my mastectomy I was back on the tennis court. When I told my surgeon, Alan Smith, about it, he said, "You can't do that!"

I said, "Too late! I already did it." I had to prove to myself that life could be normal again and playing tennis was a critical part of that life. Of course my favorite saying at the tennis court was, "If something bounces on the court and it's not yellow, for goodness sake, please don't hit it." A little humor goes a long way when you're wearing a prosthesis the size of a 38 double D. It sure made my tennis game interesting!

I thought I handled my mastectomy surgery quite well, although I wondered what I could ever put it my bra to match a 38 double D. I felt so lopsided and abnormal. I thought that anyone who looked at me could immediately tell I had lost a breast. I felt so alone, with no one to ask what they did and how they handled it. I couldn't wait for the day when my surgery healed enough to allow me to start using a prosthesis. I wasn't sure about reconstruction at that time so I decided to wait until my treatment was completed.

Throughout my years as a musician, my well endowed breasts had always been the center of attention. Men would approach the bandstand and say, "How are they -- er I mean how are you?" After all those years of people talking to my chest, they would now actually look me in the eye. What a positive change!

The thought of chemotherapy terrified me. Was it painful? Would my hair fall out immediately? Would I be sick all the time?

My first treatment was a nightmare. Fear made me sick as a dog. Before my next round of chemo I asked about the pills I was given before the actual treatment began. When the nurse told me about the tranquilizers, anti-nausea drugs, etc., I asked if I had to take them? I never was very good at taking medicine. Startled by my question, she said, "You always have a choice." So I chose not to take them and to have my treatment "cold turkey." Don't get me wrong. I had all the prescriptions filled and in my medicine cabinet. But I would be the one to decide whether I needed to take them or not.

I suddenly felt alive again. I had made a choice. What a wonderful feeling to know you have some say-so in your treatment. I was determined to tough it out with a smile on my face and found chemo was tolerable. It was certainly no fun, but I was determined to do whatever it took to survive.

I came into the treatment room armed with the latest jokes and proceeded to keep everybody laughing. I always made sure I had makeup on and wore bright colors. I wasn't going anywhere. If they wanted me, they'd have to shoot me. And I'd go down kicking and fighting. I was never going to be a victim. I chose to be victorious.

In a brief moment of insanity in 1994, I decided to run for the Florida Senate against a 16-year Republican incumbent. I, of course, ran as the lifelong Democrat I've always been. Well everyone knows what happened to the Democrats in 1994. Absolutely nothing! It was a Republican sweep.

I really loved campaigning but I hated the politics of it. It proved to be a dirty rotten business where the candidate with the most money always seemed to win. I remember the day after qualifying for the Senate race, I was being interviewed by my first special interest group. Right out of the gate, I faced a solid Republican group who lobbied on behalf of land developers. Being a known environmentalist and Democrat, I knew I didn't stand a chance of getting their money or their endorsement. What I didn't expect was their blatant discrimination against a cancer survivor.

One of the first questions I was asked was, "As a victim of cancer, Ms. de Córdova-Hanks. . ." I immediately put my hand up signaling stop, and said, "Excuse me, sir. I don't allow my name, and the words cancer and victim to be used in the same sentence."

He looked at me for a moment and changed his tactic. He said, "Do you think with your medical history, you should be running for public office?"

I looked him straight in the eye and said, "Have you checked my opponent's prostate lately? As a matter of fact gentlemen, many of you may be sitting on some very large problems you're not aware of."

The rest is history. I didn't get their endorsement but I got their respect and that was all I was really interested in.

During the campaign all candidates took part in something called Politics in the Park. It was an evening where all the candidates came to Metropolitan Park in Jacksonville and answered questions from the public. I had no idea what a big deal this evening was. I remember standing behind my table with a small amount of campaign literature, all by myself, watching my opponent enter with a whole cadre of people wearing red, white and blue hats and waving American flags. I never felt more alone than I did that very moment.

What amazed me, however, was the number of people who came up to me and told me what a difference I had made in their lives or the lives of their loved ones. Some of them reminded me that I always kept them laughing or singing in the chemo treatment room. I sure was glad I lost that election. I was right where I wanted to be. Carrying the gift of survivorship to others.

But back in 1986, I was still struggling with the fact that I had breast cancer. How could it have happened to me, a person with no family history and no apparent risk factors other than the fact that I had no biological children? Now I know that the biggest risk is just being a woman. There's no rhyme or reason to this disease. It doesn't matter how old you are, what color or creed you are or how much money you have in the bank. Breast cancer is not a bigot. It can strike any woman at any time.

Statistics show that every three minutes a woman is diagnosed with breast cancer and every 12 minutes a woman dies of breast cancer. More than 200,000 women are diagnosed each and every year. In my Bosom Buddies groups, very few of us have any of the known risk factors. How can you fight a disease when you have no idea what causes it? Or how to cure it? And that hasn't changed much in 20 years.

I learned very quickly that fear and ignorance of the disease are the enemy and that survival is real. I didn't know anyone who had breast cancer (or at least who would admit it) and I had no idea of what questions to ask or what my options were. Thank God I have a wonderful oncologist who took the time to encourage me to learn about the disease and become an active partner in decisions that would ultimately affect my whole life. Most of all, he taught me that it was okay to ask questions and to demand answers.

Dr. Tom Marsland has been a blessing in my life over my many years as a survivor. We have served as panelists together on legislative issues and once spoke as a team on how to communicate with your doctor. I think our teamwork helped enhance my survival. What more could you ask for from a doctor?

I began to think how wonderful it would be to have someone to talk to who had been through the breast cancer experience before. In 1986, there were no breast cancer support groups in Jacksonville, so I decided to educate myself about the disease as well as I could and I sort of made a silent pact with God. Boy, I sure felt funny asking God for "the big one," so I compromised. I told God if I survived, I would promise to reach out to help other women through the cancer experience. When the walls didn't come tumbling down and there were no loud claps of thunder, I decided we had struck a bargain and went about upholding my end of it.

What an overwhelming task. I was having major problems of my own. The magazine in Jacksonville that had hired me as editor closed and my insurance benefits were slowly going down the tube. I found myself out of work for more than a year with no health insurance and still dealing with treatment for my advanced cancer. I tried really hard to focus on positives during this trying time and, faced with spare time for the first time in years, I started to reach out to others.

8

Jerry's Story . . .

From Dinner to Detection

On the trip south to Cocoa Beach I told myself not to be too disappointed if Bobbi de Córdova didn't show up. After all, she didn't know what I looked like either. And even if she did, what if the night was a total disaster and we really didn't hit it off? Make the best of it, I told myself. By the same time the next day I'd be on my way back to Jacksonville and Bubba.

I didn't arrive in Cocoa Beach until after 5 o'clock and as soon as I got to the home of my friend Ed Bramlitt I decided to call the Holiday Inn and see if a Bobbi de Córdova had checked in. When she answered the phone I was so shocked I almost forgot to ask her room number.

When the time came, I drove to the motel and suddenly I was standing in front of the door to her room. What if. . . , I thought. What if. . . ? It was exactly 7 p.m. I took a deep breath and knocked on the door. In the wildest stretches of my imagination, I never anticipated the Bobbi de Córdova who answered the door. She was nearly as tall as I was and her brown hair was shorter than mine and accented by a small white birthmark right in the very front. She wore long, gold earrings, and a low cut, form fitting, black jumpsuit. And the sexiest pair of high heeled shoes I'd ever seen.

At Bernard's Surf I couldn't take my eyes off her. I had tried to prepare myself for every contingency but I never dreamed Bóbbi de Cordova would look like *this*. Normally, I like to think of myself as a fairly good conversationalist but I was so tense I could hardly speak.

After 15 or 20 minutes of very stilted talk, Bobbi asked, "Do you mind if I smoke?"

"Oh, no, not at all," I gushed. "Please go right ahead," I said as I groped in my pocket for my own pack of L&Ms. The tension evaporated in a puff of smoke. We had something in common. We were sinners of equal rank.

We had another round of drinks and we laughed and we talked -- two total strangers with nothing in common and everything to share. Bobbi originally was from New York City. For 25 years she had been a professional musician, singing and playing bass for a jazz group that toured this country, South America and Europe. I was from a steel city in eastern Pennsylvania and had spent my life as a newspaperman and public relations consultant. All my traveling had been in the other direction, to Japan, Hawaii and Viet Nam.

We ordered a third round of drinks, and we ate and then we laughed and talked our way through some of Cocoa Beach's night spots.

When it was time for the evening to end, I took Bobbi back to her room and kissed her on the forehead! As soon as I got in the car I realized how absolutely stupid that was. So I went back and knocked on her door and suggested we have breakfast a few hours later.

Breakfast was as much fun as the night had been and before we drove off in opposite directions, I asked her if she'd be willing to come to Jacksonville some time. (After all, she still had to take the Bubba test.)

I was in such a dream world I still can't remember the drive home. Bubba met me at the door and I told him everything that happened, except the part where Bobbi had told me that she had two dogs, a dachshund named B.C. and a poodle named Che. I couldn't see any reason to prejudice the judge before he had a chance to render his verdict. I shouldn't have worried.

A few weeks later Bobbi came to visit and the instant she spotted Bubba she got down on the carpet on her hands and knees and started making these funny noises, which sort of sounded like, "brooky brooky." Bubba went absolutely nuts. He couldn't get enough of this strange and wonderful creature.

The rest of the year was a blur. At least once a month, and sometimes more often, I'd drive to Miami for the weekend and on another weekend Bobbi would fly to Jacksonville.

One time we spent a weekend in Everglades City--Florida's Last Frontier, and for good reason. We were accompanied by a tropical depression and greeted by a billion mosquitoes. It poured the entire time we were there. . . and we had a wonderful time together.

Another time I talked a friend of mine at NASA into two press passes so that Bobbi and I could "cover" the first launch of the space shuttle for *The Florida Restaurateur*. My friend suggested I was stretching our friendship to the limit with this piece of absurdity but he slipped me the passes anyway. Bobbi had never seen a launch up close and we both reveled in the excitement and all of the pre- and post-launch parties in Cocoa Beach.

After nine or ten months, Bobbi and I concluded that we might enjoy more time together with a huge saving in travel expenses if we were married. It would soon be two years since Sally had died.

Bobbi and I thought it might be ecumenical if we were married in a service jointly conducted by an Episcopal priest and a Jewish rabbi. Father Riley was all for it but even with his help we could not find a single rabbi in Jacksonville who would go along with the idea.

Father Riley solved the problem. "Get me a yarmulke to wear on my head and a Hebrew prayer book and I'll perform the service in my study. Also get a glass to stomp on at the end of the ceremony in the Jewish tradition."

So that's what we did and for more than four years life was wonderful. We went everywhere and did everything together. We traveled to the Ozarks in Arkansas so Bobbi and Dad could get to know each other and Bobbi could fall in love with Eureka Springs. We visited relatives of mine in northwestern Pennsylvania and relatives of Bobbi in New York City and South Florida. And we made several trips to the University of the South at Sewanee, Tennessee, where J.R. was in college. Bobbi and my former wife Linda became friends and jointly produced J.R.'s post-graduation party at the Monteagle Assembly, near Sewanee.

Then one Sunday afternoon, after playing three sets of tennis in 90-degree heat, we returned home and decided to take a nap. When we awoke, Bobbi said, "Touch my breast right here. It feels like there's a rock inside."

My mind began to swirl and the calendar began reeling backward to a Sunday afternoon six years before when Sally had whispered, "Please don't be upset but I'm going to call a doctor tomorrow. There's something wrong with my back and the pain is almost more than I can bear." We had just finished playing three sets of tennis and had come home and taken a nap. It was the first time she had mentioned the pain.

9

Bobbi's Story...

Bosom Buddies on the Road

When I think back over the time when I was first diagnosed, what stands out most in my memory was the terrible feeling of isolation. I desperately needed other women to talk to, especially those who had been diagnosed with breast cancer and lived to talk about it. I felt like cancer was a death sentence. Now I know it's a life sentence. From that moment of diagnosis for the rest of your life, you feel like you're joined at the hip to your doctor (or doctors).

Another interesting aspect of my cancer journey was that it seemed to suddenly turn some friends into acquaintances and many acquaintances into friends. I found out quickly that a lot of people just couldn't handle my diagnosis. Maybe it hit too close to home. Maybe they were afraid they'd be next. Whatever it was, it certainly lived up to the saying, "Fair weather friends." What it did do was make me learn to love my new hometown and the wonderful caring neighbors on Woodward Avenue in Jacksonville. I've never been on so many prayer lists or had so many people pulling for me. For someone who grew up in the concrete jungle of New York, it was a welcome change.

During my treatment, I went into the room for chemotherapy with an attitude of wanting them to give me their best shot because I'd do anything to live. The doctors and nurses noticed my positive attitude and little by little began asking me if I would mind talking with other newly diagnosed women. I sort of had a buddy system going.

When my treatment was over, I suddenly felt like I had lost my security blanket. As long as I was actively doing something about my cancer, I felt like I was winning the battle. Left on my own with just a bottle of Tamoxifen wasn't the same as seeing those chemicals going into my body, killing the cancer. I visualized the chemo as little men gobbling up the bad cells and leaving the good ones. Little did I know that the chemo would take a lifetime toll on my body. But at that very moment, it was all I had.

When the day of my final treatment came, I was elated but I still had that nagging doubt of what if the chemo didn't kill what I call the "travelers and floaters" -- the microscopic bits of cells that might have escaped. Fear gave me insomnia. Insomnia gave me aches and pains. Every time I had a pain anywhere in my body, the red flag of fear went up the flagpole.

It was just around this time that I applied for a job in the public affairs department of Florida Community College at Jacksonville. I had been out of work for almost two years and had almost given up on ever finding another job, especially a challenging and creative one. I had been the frontrunner for so many jobs in the communications field, only to be let down time and time again. I began to lose confidence and thought it was me until I had a heart-to-heart talk with the vice president of a local head-hunter firm. She told me of the hidden discrimination against cancer survivors and how many employers were afraid to hire survivors because of what it might do to their insurance premiums, plus many other factors, including not believing cancer survivors could still be productive workers.

I was stunned. I asked her how these people found out about my cancer only to learn that we really have no privacy where our medical records are concerned. All someone needs is our social security number and they can call the Medical Information Bureau and find out our complete medical history. They can also find out about your credit rating at the same time. I felt like I was living in a foreign land where big brother was watching. I just couldn't believe it. This was long before the birth of the Americans with Disabilities Act. Cancer survivors had very little protection against that kind of discrimination in the late 1980s.

When the telephone call came from Ann Tillinghast, director of public affairs for the college, telling me the job was mine, I burst into tears. It was three months from the day I applied for the job. I thought it had gone by the wayside just like all the other jobs I applied for. As I sent up a silent prayer of thanks, I knew from that moment on, I would be the best employee the college ever had. I would work harder than anyone else and would always give 150 percent. Ann was very supportive. I was so happy to have the job that I was super enthusiastic about every project (which probably drove everybody else nuts). Ann used to call me "flamboyant" and said eventually people would get used to me and just say, "That's Bobbi."

When I looked like I was feeling overwhelmed, she'd say, "We've really been burning the candle at both ends lately -- let's take a couple of hours off and play." We developed a friendship that lasted long after she retired. When I won the college's Wellness Award for never missing a day of work for a year, I accepted it proudly and loudly on behalf of all cancer survivors.

As the community college's news bureau manager, I had my finger on the pulse of the community. I had a feel for what services were needed and were unmet. The first thing I did was approach the dean of lifelong learning to ask if I could offer a "course" on surviving cancer for the women in the community who were struggling with the emotional ravages of breast cancer. Thankfully, I received a great deal of support from Carol Miner, president of the College's Open Campus, and the seed for Bosom Buddies was planted. Carol was the first person to give us a home and I'll always be grateful for that. I already had a good buddy system going and what better name for a breast cancer support and education program than Bosom Buddies?

As we began to get a lot of media coverage, I was startled to find out that this was a threat to a well known cancer agency. I was outraged. After all, aren't we all out to help the people suffering from the same disease? Was there actually competition in helping people? I guess I was naive. But when letters to the editor and to the president of the college began to surface, I quickly learned that cancer is big business. No wonder there's no cure! They began by asking for my "credentials." I told them I had earned an "M.S." and a "Ph.D." In my case, that stood for "master of survival" and "patient hasn't died." Can you think of better credentials? I believe what really upset them was that I was offering services free of charge and accomplishing with almost no money what they should have been doing with their endless fundraising. What an eye-opener that was! That was in 1988 and Bosom Buddies is still going strong.

Bosom Buddies became a force to be reckoned with. We armed newly diagnosed women with information and education that would help them become active members of their health care team. We taught them their rights as patients and how to look for the best doctors when assembling that team. They also learned to look for compassionate doctors who would be confident enough to answer the questions they asked, and the importance of second opinions and third opinions, if necessary. As a grassroots group that was not beholden to the medical community, we could have been models for that popular T-shirt that said, "No Fear." I think that once you face your own mortality and do battle with a life-threatening illness, everything else pales in comparison.

Our "buddie" system became widely known. We tried to match women with "buddies" by age, marital status, common interests and neighborhoods. We took pride in the fact that this was a special sisterhood which welcomed anyone with the common bond of breast cancer, regardless of race, creed, socioeconomic level, or sexual preference. We were one for all and all for one.

And what a zany group of women we were. There were members like Margaret Swartley, whom I called "legs," because she didn't work and did a lot of running around on behalf of Bosom Buddies. And the gracious Brenda Murray. We were like ham hocks and matzo balls, Brenda coming from Georgia and me from New York. What a pair we made. She is a true Steel Magnolia, having been diagnosed with breast cancer and Hodgkin's Disease at the same time. There was Terry Thompson and her children, Kelly and Mathew, who stuffed envelopes and educational packets on their off-hours from school and very often helped to staff our table at health fairs. Kelly and Mathew became our first Junior Volunteers of the Year. What treasures they were. Edith Ibach and her late husband Rudy, made wooden salad bowls and sold them to benefit Bosom Buddies. And Barbara Holland brought her cosmetics and colors to meetings to help us look good and feel better about ourselves. And there were many others who followed in their footsteps and became such an important part of my life.

I'll never forget Coleen Choley, who thought up our first National Cancer Survivors Day T-shirt slogan, "Not Extinct -- Six Million Survivor-Sauruses." When we learned that Coleen's cancer had recurred and the prognosis was grim, we had a pajama party in her honor and we laughed and cried together for this young mother and the small children she would leave behind.

Having a full-time job apart from Bosom Buddies, I relied heavily on volunteers. We held garage sales that were the talk of the neighborhood. No one could believe these women hugging and laughing were cancer survivors. We traveled together to conferences on planes, reading aloud from "Hormones from Hell" and flying our Bosom Buddies banner. By the time our flight came to an end, the other passengers were toasting us with champagne. We were incorrigible.

We even rented a van one time to drive to a conference in Charlotte, North Carolina with a magnetic sign on the van that read "Bosom Buddies -- Charlotte or Bust!" We had all the other cars on the road honking and saluting us. I had written a rap song for the group and we jumped out of our van in matching Bosom Buddies T-shirts, carrying pom-poms and rapping away. We even made national TV with that episode.

Most of all, we became soul sisters. Friendships were forged that will last forever. We showed the world that we were more than cancer survivors. We were women who laughed and cried, had jobs and families and bled for each other when one of us died. When we lost our beloved Marva Holston at the age of 34, it was Bosom Buddies and their spouses who took turns caring for this incredibly courageous young African-American 24 hours a day so she wouldn't be alone. Race never entered the picture. It was her wish to be surrounded by Bosom Buddies when her time came to leave this earth and we honored that wish to the very end. I believe there's a special band of angels with butterflies on their wings, our Bosom Buddies, looking down on us from above telling us everything is OK up there. Every time I see a butterfly in my garden, I stop for a few moments knowing it just may be the spirit of one of our Bosom Buddies paying me a visit. And I smile.

As time rolled by and my involvement grew, I realized how little information was out there for survivors. I also realized how important cancer research is, but I knew that without quality of life and good productive life, we might not be around to benefit from the research. How could I take my involvement one step further?

10

Jerry's Story...

The Little Old Lady in Vancouver

Being a cancer caregiver is no easier the second time around. Everything is new and different. I was as scared over what I felt in Bobbi's breast as she was and I feared the worst.

Several years ago when I joined Bobbi as a public speaker on the subjects of cancer survivorship and cancer caregiving I put together a presentation called, "10 Tips on How to Be a Good Cancer Caregiver." It didn't work and I tossed it out. Individual situations vary too much.

The best I can ever hope to do when I'm speaking with Bobbi is to share my personal experiences -- the good ones and the bad -- and hope that among those who hear me will be some who can relate to my stories and be filled anew with hope and optimism. If nothing else, I hope that there will be at least a few who will discover that they're not the only ones who have ever broken down in tears, or become so angry and frustrated that they have looked at their image in the mirror and screamed, "Why me?", forgetting entirely that the person they are caring for didn't exactly volunteer to be diagnosed with cancer.

Being a cancer caregiver is not an easy job. But it has its moments of joy.

The first speaking engagement I went on with Bobbi was to Vancouver, British Columbia, where we had been invited by the British Columbia-Yukon Chapter of the Canadian Breast Cancer Foundation. We had just finished speaking at a fund-raising luncheon in the huge ballroom of the Hyatt Regency in downtown Vancouver. The program was over and everyone was slowly heading toward the exits. Some people had come up to talk with Bobbi and me when out of the corner of my eye I saw this tiny lady fighting against the crowd as if she were trying to get to where we were.

A few moments later she was standing right in front of me. She could not have been five feet tall or weighed 85 pounds. She also must have been at least 85 years old -- and she had the most beautiful smile I think I've ever seen.

"Mr. Hanks, Mr. Hanks," she said, looking up at me, "I just wanted to tell you how interested I was in what you said."

I was thrilled. But before I could thank her she added, "I wrote down every single word you said."

"You did?" I exclaimed in astonishment.

"Yes, look," she said, and she pulled out a steno pad and started flipping through the pages, each one of them covered with strange looking Oriental symbols. I didn't know you could take shorthand in Korean or Japanese or Chinese or whatever I was looking at. I was totally fascinated and I asked if she was a caregiver.

"Oh, yes," she said proudly and went on to explain that she lived in a high rise building on the edge of downtown Vancouver in what sounded to me like an assisted living facility.

"Another lady who lives on the same floor was diagnosed with breast cancer," the tiny lady in front of me explained. "She doesn't have any close friends or relatives in this part of Canada. And I'm really not very busy myself any more, so I asked if she'd let me be her caregiver."

I stood there looking at her and I was seized with the urge to call everyone who was still in the ballroom back to their seats. They had just heard the wrong person talk about caregiving. I would like to have joined them in the audience and heard more from this tiny lady with the beautiful smile.

I like to tell the story about her for several reasons.

For one, it speaks with such quiet eloquence about the limitless love that exists between a cancer survivor and a cancer caregiver. It is a love that knows no bounds--nor should it ever.

Another reason I like to tell the story is that it reminds us that cancer caregivers, like cancer survivors, come in all sizes and shapes and sexes and, yes, from all ethnic origins. So often we think of a husband caring for a wife or a wife for a husband, or a brother for a sister or vice versa, or a son or daughter caring for a parent, or, sadly, parents caring for a small child. And then sometimes. . .sometimes. . .it's simply a friend . . . caring for a friend.

And, finally, I like to tell the story because it tells us that we never really know when we are going to be called on to be a caregiver. It might be tomorrow, or next week, or next month, or next year. Or maybe it will be when we are 85 years old. I know I never expected to become a cancer caregiver for a third time when Bobbi was diagnosed again, this time for thyroid cancer.

When the time comes, you're never really prepared. And by then it's too late to ask, "Why?" or "Why me?" The only valid questions left to ask are, "What do I do now?" and "How can I help?"

11

Bobbi's Story . . .

Survivor --
From the Moment of Diagnosis

As time rolled by and my involvement in survivorship grew, I realized how little information was available about life after cancer. I knew the value of cancer research, but I also realized that without quality of life, we might not be around to benefit from the research.

As Bosom Buddies grew and I became more involved in being a consumer of cancer survivorship, I learned of an organization founded by 25 survivors in Albuquerque, New Mexico in 1986. That's when the National Coalition for Cancer Survivorship came into my life and my life changed dramatically.

NCCS reinforced the fact that survival is real and that fear and ignorance of the disease are the enemies. The NCCS definition of a survivor includes anyone with a history of cancer, from the point of diagnosis for the balance of life, whether that is for months, years or decades. When I attended my first national assembly in 1988, I was in awe of the quality of leadership that came from NCCS. I was overwhelmed to be among hundreds of other cancer survivors and to experience an instant bond. I was impressed by the lack of self-pity and the positive feelings reinforced by the group. I found a second family. I found hope. I found joy. And I received a great education.

I now know that more than 10 million people are alive today in the United States, after a diagnosis of cancer, most of them survivors of five years or more. I learned that we, as survivors, should have the right to assurance of lifelong medical care, have the right to the pursuit of happiness and to be free of the stigma of cancer. I learned we need to advocate to have the right to equal job opportunities and to have health insurance coverage regardless of pre-existing conditions. Most of all, I learned to be proud to be a cancer survivor.

While I learned about "survivor pride," I also learned the realities of living with a cancer diagnosis and the often hidden discriminations we face. I jumped right into the survivorship movement, serving four years on the board of directors of the National Coalition for Cancer Survivorship as its communications chair. What an eye-opener! Those were some of the most informative years for me. Who would ever think that a Brooklyn born bass player would ever speak at congressional hearings? What in life had prepared me to fight for a cause I so deeply believed in? I guess when you're determined to beat the odds, you'll do anything to help make a difference for those who will ultimately follow in your footsteps. And follow they did -- about 200,000 women plus each year.

We wrote position papers and press releases, signed NCCS' Ribbon of Hope and marched on Washington. We were drawn together to conquer cancer, united against this faceless enemy. As the late Natalie Davis Spingarn said in the title of her first book, we were "Hanging in There -- Living Well on Borrowed Time."

With Bosom Buddies in tow, we traveled around the country to NCCS conferences, preaching the gospel of survivorship and defying anyone to call us victims. We shared hugs and tears and our emotions overwhelmed us as we swayed to the beat of a gospel choir at the end of conferences. Time might run out for some of us, but we'd never allow anyone to say we lost the battle.

In the early days of my involvement with NCCS, my heroes were founders and survivors like Dr. Fitzhugh Mullan, first president of NCCS; Catherine Logan Carrillo, first executive director and founder of People Living Through Cancer; Susan Leigh, RN, BSN, Vietnam veteran and a past president of NCCS; Barbara Hoffman, general counsel for NCCS, working to stop discrimination against cancer survivors in the workplace long before the Americans With Disabilities Act, and the late Natalie Davis Spingarn, writer and first editor of the NCCS newsletter. What role models!

I remember Susan Leigh, a survivor of Hodgkin's Disease, breast cancer and bladder cancer saying, "After the third diagnosis, cancer is just an inconvenience." You can't imagine what those words did for me, especially after my own second diagnosis in December 1999. I remember the first book on survivorship that I read, "Vital Signs: A Young Doctor's Struggle with Cancer," by Fitzhugh Mullan, and the enormous pride I felt in knowing him and serving in the survivorship movement with him. He's still in the public health field working as a clinical professor of pediatrics and public health at George Washington University and still looking out for the well-being of others in his "spare" time.

These people were, and are, the voice of cancer survivors everywhere, standing up for our collective rights while mapping and cultivating our common ground. How proud I felt being a part of this vital organization, now being spearheaded by two-time survivor Ellen Stovall, executive director at that time, and Susan Sher, survivor and then deputy director -- two women whose friendship I cherish.

I also learned that we are not alone in our quest for survivorship. Cancer is a disease that involves the entire family. People always notice someone in a wheelchair, but how many notice the person pushing the chair? The invisible survivors. This really touched home when my mother

Florence was diagnosed with breast cancer on her 83rd birthday and when my younger sister Adrienne was diagnosed in December 2001. I was now the invisible survivor and I experienced the helplessness you feel watching someone you love face this diagnosis. Both of them had been by my side every step of the way from the moment I was diagnosed and through all the following challenges. Now it was my turn to be there for them. It gave me the opportunity to pass along the vital knowledge I had gained through my own experience with cancer.

Every June when we celebrate National Cancer Survivors Day, we honor these invisible survivors -- our families, our friends, our coworkers and most of all our health care partners. But we cannot leave the responsibility for our survival in their hands alone. We must educate ourselves and advocate for ourselves. We must learn the role of a survivor. We have to learn to look for the best doctors, the best treatments and to surround ourselves with those who believe in survivorship. Why is it that after you're diagnosed, people love to come out of the woodwork and tell you all these dreadful stories like, "My Aunt Sadie in Pittsburgh had breast cancer. She was sick 24 hours a day during chemo. . . and then she died!"

Statistics now show that one out of every three families will be touched by cancer. The good news is that there's great life after cancer. It makes you stop and smell the roses. It gives you an opportunity to tell your family and friends how much you love them. It gives you a chance to make a difference in the world. How lucky I am to be a survivor. It's been such a positive force in my life.

I've learned so much since my cancer journey began in 1986. I've learned to go to Congress and fight for our rights. I've even learned to use cancer when I need it. I figure if I have to deal with it, I'll use it to my advantage. I remember when I was follically challenged (also known as being bald) and they tried to bump me off a plane from Washington, D. C. to Jacksonville. I just stood there at the counter, whipped off my wig and false eyelashes, and the next thing I knew I was sitting in first class and drinking champagne while winging my way back home.

All survivors live on a seesaw. Over the years we've been told silicone implants were safe, then that was questionable, now doctors are using them once again. Node negative women didn't need chemo, then they did and now they don't. If we had chemo they didn't treat us with radiation therapy. Now they believe it would help to enhance our survival.

Not only do we have to live with a life-threatening disease, we have to live with all the uncertainty that surrounds it while dedicated researchers probe for new and better drugs, therapies and treatment protocols. For those of us who are survivors, life becomes a crap shoot. Who lives and who doesn't? And who can really predict one's chances? While we may live with uncertainty, we pray every day that those same researchers find the answers during our lifetime.

12

Jerry's Story . . .

How to Be a Good Caregiver

Much has been written and said about being a good cancer caregiver and most of it I agree with, based on my experiences with Sally and Bobbi.

Certainly I agree that it's important to have faith in a power greater than your own. I'm not theologically qualified to preach a sermon on the subject but I'm sure everyone knows exactly what I'm talking about. I'll add this one thought, however, and that simply is that as a caregiver you may reach a point where your faith is *all* you have. And that faith can be like a rock of stability in a raging torrent of emotions.

I also agree that it's important to be an informed consumer and to know all you can not only about caregiving but also about the disease itself and its diagnosis, treatment protocols and medications that help the survivor with treatment side effects. Ignorance breeds fear. Education fosters understanding and hope, and helps you share in the treatment and emotions of the person entrusted to your care.

But an equally important reason to know all you can about cancer is to prepare yourself for the role of patient advocate.

It's easy to tell yourself you're not qualified to fill this role and serve as spokesperson. But there will be times when the person you're caring for simply is not up to the task--physically, mentally or emotionally--and the job is yours whether you want it or not.

A sportswriter many years ago is said to have asked John Brodie, the ace quarterback of the San Francisco 49ers, why it was he who performed such a mundane task as holding the football for point after touchdown conversions. Brodie's answer: "If I don't hold it, the ball will fall over."

That's about the way it is with being a patient advocate. You may think you're not the one who should do it, or you can't afford to take the time off from work, or any of 10 other reasons, but the bottom line is that if you don't do it the job won't get done.

And when your turn comes, and it's time to accompany the person in your care to see the doctor, be prepared. Write down your questions, and those of the survivor, ahead of time and when the two of you face the doctor make absolutely sure the doctor answers every single question you have. . . in language that you can understand. And do not leave until you have received an intelligent, and intelligible, answer to every question on your list.

Most doctors I have met say they welcome questions and, more than that, they welcome an advocate who comes along with the patient. Patients under stress have a very human tendency to hear only what they want to hear and to ask only those questions they hope will elicit an encouraging response.

If the doctor is not as "consumer oriented" as you might like and rebuffs your questions, press on. You don't have to be obnoxious, but you might find it helpful to remind the doctor that it's not his or her life that's in peril but the life of the person you're caring for. And if the doctor still doesn't have the time, or the professional knowledge and courtesy, to answer your questions it just may be time to find another doctor.

Tough task? You bet! But being a cancer caregiver can be a tough job, second only to being a cancer survivor. And you don't score any points if the ball falls over.

Another thing I agree with about cancer caregiving is that it's important to participate in a support group, something like the Bosom Buddies support group that Bobbi founded for survivors in Jacksonville and others that have sprung up around the country.

There's strength to be gained in discovering that you're not the first person who has felt the frustration, anger, despair -- and sometimes joy -- that comes with being a caregiver. And there's a certain feeling of goodness that comes with sharing your experiences and providing an understanding ear to others who may have just entered the ranks.

But having said all that, let me be honest and say that I think participating in a support group seems to be easier for a woman than it is for a man.

Call me sexist if you like, but from the time we are little boys, members of the male sex are trained to hide their emotions. What's the first thing we're told when we take a tumble and skin our knee? "Come on now, don't cry. Be a little man. Mommy will put a Band-Aid on it and then you can go on back out and play."

Then when we get older we start playing sports and we're taught to "play through the pain," "suck it up," "tough it out," and "don't let the other team know they got to you, kid."

I went to high school in Bethlehem, Pennsylvania, and was the starting goalkeeper on the soccer team in my junior year. We were playing at Upper Darby, near Philadelphia, when I scooped up a ball in a wild melee and tried to get it out of the goal box by flinging it to safety. When I threw it, my thumb snagged on somebody's jersey and snapped it back all the way to my wrist.

I crumpled to the ground in pain. Meanwhile the game was still going on. Dick Van Atta, one of our fullbacks, saw me on the ground and yelled, "Jerry, are you OK?" When I couldn't answer, he yelled again, "See if you can get up. We'll try to keep the ball away from you." Somehow I crawled to my feet, clutching my hand and wrist, which already were beginning to swell.

At halftime, I tried to talk to the coach but he was engrossed in trying to inspire our forwards to score a goal or two. Our "trainer" was a year ahead of me in school and I knew it wouldn't do any good to talk to him.

I went back out for the second half not knowing exactly how I was going to protect the goal, since the pain eliminated any possibility of me catching the ball with my hands. Our fullbacks, Dick and Lawrence Meixell, played the game of their lives for the next 45 minutes and what few balls got past them I was able to kick to safety. We won the game, 2-0.

As we were leaving the field, here comes Bill Stark, our coach, heading straight for me. He was an aging, grayhaired Scotsman of the old school, and the first thing he said to me was, "Now let me take a look at that hand and let's see if we can get some ice on it."

Then he looked me straight in the eye and wrapped one of his massive arms around my shoulders and said, "You showed a lot of guts, laddie."

It was one of the proudest moments of my young life and it taught me a lesson I needed to learn, that sometimes you grit your teeth and you really do play through the pain for the sake of your team, or your squad or sometimes, even, your office.

Others have learned the same lesson in far more important, heroic and dramatic ways. Unfortunately, all of the good that comes out of this hard-earned lesson seems to be matched by the stoic belief that you should never express the pain you are feeling or let down your guard and ask for help.

Women seem to do much better at overcoming this false sense of bravado than men. What about me? How have I changed as a three-time cancer caregiver? Not much. I'm still the John Wayne, macho-type who'll tell you everything is fine when inside my heart is breaking.

But I'll stop anything I'm doing to help someone else -- if only they'll ask me. After Sally died, I promised myself I'd do all I could to help other men who were going through what I had endured.

About two months later the wife of a friend of mine was diagnosed with cancer and the prognosis was not encouraging. I asked my friend one day if I could be of help. "I've walked in your shoes. I know how it feels inside. If you'd ever like to talk, please let me know, day or night."

He looked at me with tears in his eyes and said, "Jerry, you don't know how much that means to me."

But he never called.

Over the next year so, I made the same offer six or seven times to others, always with the same result. In my heart I knew why no one called. But the offer still remains open.

What's the best advice? Find a support group, or start one of your own, and become an active participant even if it means letting your guard down.

Now let me tell you a couple of things about cancer caregiving that you're not likely to read or hear anyplace else.

13

Bobbi's Story...

The Faces of Courage

I've always wondered what other people think about cancer survivors. Of course, part of the public's misconception or perception is fueled by the media. They're always looking for the worst-case scenario. I remember during all of our National Cancer Survivors Day celebrations in Jacksonville that newspaper photographers and television reporters weren't too interested in healthy looking people laughing and enjoying themselves. They usually spent their time looking for someone without hair or someone in a wheelchair . . . and if they were hooked up to an oxygen tank, or looked to be about 15 years old, so much the better.

Now don't get me wrong. There are some wonderful journalists who are truly dedicated to the plight of people battling cancer. But that's not what sells newspapers or puts television stations at the top of the rating charts. I especially remember one year when I desperately tried to get media coverage for our Survivors Day event only to be told that, "Survivorship is overdone. It's old hat. Tell me your worst case scenario." My answer was, "My worst-case scenario would be being interviewed by you." Believe me, they still don't get the message.

Every time I make a television appearance or participate in a radio talk show, the reporter or host always says, "Funny, you don't look like a cancer survivor!" What would they see if they peered through the window of any Bosom Buddies meeting? They'd see women laughing, joking, hugging, and, yes, sometimes sharing tears . . . women getting on with life, breasts or no breasts. They'd see "breast friends."

The late Natalie Davis Spingarn wrote a sequel to her first book that I talked about earlier, "Hanging in There . . . Living Well on Borrowed Time," which is a classic on cancer survivorship that everyone should read. The sequel was called, "The New Cancer Survivors: Living with Grace, Fighting with Spirit," and how true that is.

When I founded Bosom Buddies in 1988, women were so eager to come to meetings to share stories and learn all they could from the veteran survivors. They came without preconceived ideas and were totally open to any information they could glean from others. My Bosom Buddies that followed are just the opposite. The group is made up of many more young women than ever before. They are born activists. They spend hours on the internet researching everything possible about breast cancer. They come to meetings armed with copies of all of the latest articles from the web, wanting to share information with everyone. Every evening my e-mail piles up with loving messages loaded with new information. I can just see the fingers flying over their keyboards. The messages are so bright and full of hope!

If I had had a daughter, I would have wanted her to be a combination of Jennifer Levinson, with her commitment to advocate on behalf of young breast cancer survivors, and Tammy Cross and her teenage daughter Danielle, who bring a lot of love into my life. There are so many other "buddies" who lift my spirit, like Lori Covell, our resident massage therapist who helps us to understand lymphedema and how to control it; Darlene Davenport and Stephanie Michaud, who are always willing to volunteer to hand out breast cancer awareness information at every opportunity and Linda

Cornelio, who brings us information on the latest and greatest in complementary medicine that may enhance breast cancer treatment.

And I can't help but mention Caroline Windsor, Denise Creighton and Caraline Everson, who are no longer with us, but whose courage was unbelievable.

When people ask why I'm still doing this for almost two decades, all I have to do is look at these young women for my answer. How I wish for a world where young women like these would never have to face this disease we call breast cancer. I would like to gather them all into my arms and protect them forever. I even made up a "magic wand" to use when the going gets really tough. When anyone I care about a great deal becomes very ill and tells me they don't want to die, I bring out my magic wand and tell them, "If I could wave this magic wand and make all of us well again, I would. But I can't." All I can do is hug them, love them, pray for them and be with them until they are at peace. And then go out and curse this vile disease called breast cancer.

There is such an incredible survivor-to-survivor bond. It transcends age, religion, color, social status and how much you have in the bank. Once we have walked in each other's shoes, we are bound together forever. The love and support from your family and friends is vital, but there's nothing like being able to say to someone, "Been there! Done that!" It's a great equalizer.

Now when someone says, "Funny, you don't look like a cancer survivor," I always smile, knowing that cancer survivors are everywhere, come from every walk of life and are of every imaginable color and creed. What does a cancer survivor look like? When you look at a survivor, you're looking at the face of courage, determination and hope. That's what I see when I look at a cancer survivor.

Over the years I've met some of the most courageous women imaginable . . . many of whom are carrying the gift of survivorship to the far corners of the world. All of us are committed to sharing this precious gift of life. And isn't that really what it's all about?

14

Jerry's Story...

Getting Mad and Shedding Tears

Let me tell you a couple of things about being a cancer caregiver that you may not find anywhere else.

One of them is that I think it's OK to get angry. Before anyone misunderstands what I'm saying please let me stress that I am *not* advocating violence. Nor am I suggesting that you stay mad all of the time. But every now and then. . .

There was the noon that I went to see Sally at the hospital in Jacksonville and I became incensed over the care that I did not think she was receiving. The first nurse I found, I let her have it. And I didn't spare the four-letter words. When I was done with her I found another and then another until I had wiped out the entire nursing corps in that wing of the fourth floor.

Then I went downstairs to the administrative and executive offices and started working my way up through the chain of command. When I finally ran out of people to accost, I returned to my office in the Gulf Life Building and went back to work.

A little after 5 o'clock the phone rang and it was Dr. Irvin Schneider, Sally's doctor and one of the most wonderful men I've ever met. "Jerry," he said in his very soft Southern drawl, "I understand that you were at the hospital around noon today and had a few uncomplimentary things to say to some of the members of the staff."

"Uh, that's true, Dr. Schneider," I stammered, suddenly feeling very guilty. "But I want you to understand that none of what I said was intended for you. I'm sorry if any of it spilled over. That's not what I had in mind. You know Sally and I think the world of you. What I really intended. . ."

"Jerry," Dr. Schneider interrupted, "will you please stop it? Look," he said quietly, "I just have a suspicion that one or two of those people you talked to probably deserved to hear every single word you said. And I suspect, too, that you might have had a few things building up inside that you needed to get off your chest."

There was a long silence and finally I said, "Is that all, Dr. Schneider?"

"Well," he said, "I see by the clock in my office that it's almost 5:15 and I imagine that it's about time for you to get back to the hospital and spend some time with that lovely bride of yours."

But that's not the end of the story.

Would you believe that from that day on there never again was one single problem with the care Sally received at that hospital? What I have never figured out was whether that was true because of my tirade. . .or whether Dr. Schneider had gone behind me and had a few words of his own to say.

Thirteen years later I tried somewhat the same tactic at a cancer center in Tampa. Dr. Schneider had retired and this time the patient was Bobbi. She had been operated on early that morning for thyroid cancer and then was taken to recovery while her room in the hospital was "being prepared."

When it seemed time for her to be taken to her hospital room, I was told that she would have to stay in recovery a while longer because her room was still not ready

-- even though her surgery had taken eight and one-half hours. So we waited. And waited. And waited. After two more hours I decided it was time for action. I asked the volunteer in the waiting area outside of recovery for the location of Bobbi's room and then set forth on a little journey.

When I got to the nursing station near where Bobbi's room was supposed to be, I found four nurses engaged in a full blown talkfest. I politely introduced myself and asked when I could expect my wife's room to be ready.

"We'll be getting to it very shortly, Mr. Hanks," the head nurse gushed. "We have been having one of *those* days and I'm sure you know how that goes," she added and smiled at me coyly.

"As a matter of fact," I said, "I have no idea at all how that goes. It seems quite obvious that you have no shortage of help and I see no reason why my wife's room should not be ready in 30 minutes."

Without another word or a smile I turned and went back to recovery and said that a slight misunderstanding had now been corrected and that my wife's room would be ready when she arrived.

It was.

After Bobbi was finally placed in bed and made as comfortable as possible, I decided to go to the cafeteria for something to eat. On my way past the nurse's station I nodded at the head nurse and said, "Appreciate your help."

She stared at me in icy silence.

Tactics like these aren't intended to win popularity contests. Except with the person you're caring for.

Another conclusion I've come to is that it's OK to cry. There were times when I'd leave Sally's hospital room and go out to the parking garage and sit there with the windows in the car rolled up and cry my heart out.

Every time I tell about this, someone says, "Well, did Sally ever see you cry?"

And, sadly, the answer is no. Sally never saw me cry. And I'm not sure I did the right thing. But Sally was a winner and I don't think she ever had a negative thought in her life. And I was afraid that if she saw me cry she'd think I was having negative thoughts of my own and I couldn't bear the idea of letting her down.

Even on the night before she died, Sally told me to tell the other girls in the office to get ready, that she'd be back to work the following week. And I think she truly meant it. So I choked back the tears and held her frail, little hand. And Sally never saw me cry.

For some strange reason it reminds of an interview of Johnny Unitas I once saw on television. Johnny's playing days with the Baltimore Colts were over and he was reminiscing about his career and one of the things he opined, if I remember it correctly, was that he didn't really think he'd ever played in a losing football game. The worst that ever happened, in Johnny's opinion, was that a few times the game ended before he really wanted it to. But there was never any doubt in his mind that if he'd had just a few more minutes he would have thought of something and the Colts would have won.

And that's sort of the way it was with Sally. Time ran out before she wanted it to, 311 days after being diagnosed with an advanced recurrence of ovarian cancer. But I'll tell you one thing: I never regretted a single second of those 311 days we shared together after her diagnosis.

And I'll tell you something else: I've never regretted a single second of the more than 7,300 days that Bobbi and I have shared together since her diagnosis with advanced breast cancer on May 22, 1986.

Bobbi is a winner. Sally was a winner. All cancer survivors are winners. And for those of us who are fortunate enough to be cancer caregivers, it's great to be part of a winning team.

The numbers may have increased by the time you read this, but do you realize that in this country today there are more than 10.5 million cancer survivors? And that most of them have been survivors for more than five years? And that the ranks are growing every day with discoveries of new techniques for early detection. . .new treatment protocols . . . and new research and medicines that extend survival?

Think about it. More than 10,500,000 cancer survivors. Now add just one caregiver for each survivor and you have an army of nearly 21,000,000 survivors and caregivers united in their battle against cancer. An army that doesn't know the meaning of the word defeat.

Next time you wake up in the middle of the night feeling frightened and all alone in your battle against cancer, remember that there are 21,000,000 others who at one time or another have felt just the way you do. Don't be afraid to call upon them for help. They're not only winners. . .they're also friends.

15

Bobbi's Story...

The Second Time Around

When 1999 started, I expected it to be a terrific year for me. I knew that by the end of the year I would retire from the community college, where I had been working for 13 years, and finally have the opportunity to expand Bosom Buddies to a full-time organization. For me it was to be a dream come true.

As I began planning the next step for Bosom Buddies, I had a sense of "deja vu all over again," as Yogi Berra once said, where my health was concerned. I couldn't quite put my finger on it, but I knew deep down that once again, something was seriously wrong. I had been suffering from hyperparathyroidism for quite a while. I attributed my growing fatigue and sense of malaise to that. I underwent an unsuccessful exploratory surgery to try to locate and remove the bad parathyroid gland.

The parathyroid is a tiny, pea-size gland embedded in the thyroid gland in the neck and produces a parathyroid hormone. This hormone, together with vitamin D and calcitonin (a hormone produced by the thyroid gland), controls the level of calcium in the body. This condition is most often caused by a small, benign tumor in one or more of the parathyroid glands. About 40 persons in 100,000 suffer from the disorder, which usually develops after the age of 40 and is twice as common in women as men. When you suffer from the condition, your body overproduces the parathyroid hormone and raises the level of calcium in the blood, causing hypercalcemia, which leads to osteoporosis. Instead of strengthening the bones, this actually weakens them.

In one of my routine checkups to try and get a handle on this disease, my doctor shocked me by telling me that there was a large mass in my chest that showed up during a routine chest x-ray. I should have known there was more to it when the doctor got up, took my hand and said, "I'm so very sorry." I hadn't the foggiest notion of what he meant. It had been 13 years since I was diagnosed with breast cancer. That couldn't possibly be the problem.

He immediately referred me to a surgeon and Jerry and I once again were anxiously sitting in a waiting room. I remember signing in and hearing two other women say that they had an 11 a.m. appointment with the same doctor. I asked the receptionist how three of us could have an appointment at the same time? Her answer was, "Well, we have three examining rooms." I said, "You may have three examining rooms, but you only have one doctor." That should have been a warning to me that this "clinic" didn't care how long the patients waited regardless of the seriousness of the situation.

One hour went by. Two hours went by. My name was finally called and we were taken to an examining room and told the doctor would be right with us. Another hour went by. And another hour went by. In my anxiety over the mass in my chest, I put up with the wait. At the end of four hours, I went out of the room and into the reception area only to find everyone had left. I couldn't believe it.

The clinic had a patient advocate so I headed for her office. When I told her what happened, she paged the doctor. His reason for not showing up was that when he went to my examining room, he saw that my cat scans were not ready for him to look at. I was flabbergasted. I knew that was not true. My other doctor had shown my scans to me several days before when he made the appointment for me with the surgeon.

At this point I knew I wouldn't let this doctor get anywhere near me. I called the medical records department and asked for all my records. I was going to find a doctor who cared about his or her patients. I was told I would have to wait 10 days to get my records. I told them they had 20 minutes to bring my records to me or I would stand in their lobby and repeat what had just happened to me in three languages. I'd start in English, switch to Spanish and end up in French. Considering the number of international patients the clinic had, that did the trick. Twenty-one minutes later, a sweaty volunteer came racing over and handed me an enormous stack of medical records. We left wondering where to go next.

I knew we had to find out what the mass was so I entered another local hospital to have a needle biopsy of the mass, which I had been told previously was not possible to biopsy. In my heightened sense of apprehension, I was flabbergasted when I went to sign in at the hospital only to be told I wasn't "on the list" for any procedure that day. I quickly called the office of the doctor, who had arranged this for me, to straighten everything out. By this time my nerves were raw and my usual positive attitude took a nosedive. The next thing I remembered was waking up and being told to go home and celebrate. It was just scar tissue from the advanced breast cancer. That should have been a happy ending, but unfortunately it wasn't.

My symptoms got worse and I became weaker and weaker. I was at my wit's end when Dr. Gary Bowers, a surgical oncologist who wasn't even my doctor, but was very involved in treating breast cancer patients, found a doctor in Tampa at the Moffitt Cancer Center who was considered tops in the area of head and neck surgery. Even though I wasn't his patient, Dr. Bowers gave me a referral to see Dr. Douglas Klotch. I was surprised when I called Dr. Klotch long-distance to have him call me back and talk to me for nearly half an hour. He was very positive about being able to help me so Jerry and I loaded up our conversion van and burned rubber for Tampa.

It was a very different experience to have to leave my home and all that was familiar to me. Jerry was my rock. Being the writer that he is and accustomed to interviewing people, he had prepared several pages of questions for the doctor. The doctor was new to both of us, and although we trusted Dr. Bowers' judgment, we wanted to be sure Dr. Klotch was the doctor for us. We were sure he was a good doctor, but we also had to feel comfortable with him. Much to our surprise, he answered most of the questions before we even asked them and he thought it was terrific that we had come so well prepared. I really think he enjoyed having a patient who wanted to be active in all of the decisions. Sometimes I think we expect too much from doctors when we leave the total responsibility for our care in their hands alone. It has to be a team effort. We left Tampa and returned home to prepare for the upcoming surgery and whatever might follow.

I remember telling Dr. Klotch if he saw anything suspicious while he was "in there," to remove it if I didn't need it to live. He was very upbeat and didn't seem to suspect cancer at all. He was sure my problems would be solved by the removal of the parathyroid gland alone. What was expected to be a surgery that should take a few hours at most, ended up taking eight and one-half hours. He did a thyroidectomy, parathyroidectomy, thymusectomy and removed the mass from the mediastinal area of my chest. I had the easy part. I slept through it all with no recollection of the time it took to do the surgery. Poor Jerry was the one it took a toll on. No one came out during the whole time period to let him know what was happening.

Other than the usual effects of any surgery, I felt great. It was amazing how the removal of a bad parathyroid gland can instantly make a huge difference. I was shocked when the doctor came to my room around midnight to check up on me. That was definitely a first.

I was in the hospital for the better part of a week while Jerry was staying at a motel nearby. Just before Christmas, I went home for the holidays, stitches from one ear to the other -- literally.

About 10 days later, we returned to Tampa to have the stitches removed and learn the results of the surgery. Dr. Klotch was very positive, telling me how well the surgery went when his nurse walked in with the pathology report. He took a look at it, stopped in the middle of the removal of the stitches and said, "There's cancer in three areas." That's all I remember hearing. I must have looked wild-eyed because he stood up, took my face in his hands and said, "Look at me. It's better than any kind of breast cancer. It's treatable. It's curable."

Once again I was faced with a metastatic cancer. It was in both lobes of the thyroid, the thymus gland and the mediastinum mass was malignant also. My world turned topsy-turvy again as I began part two of my cancer journey.

16

Jerry's Story . . .

Fighting the Good Fight

Every now and then someone asks me what I think was the big difference between Sally and Bobbi. What I always suspect they're asking is why Bobbi has survived for so much longer in the hope that they may discover some hidden secret for survival.

Oh, that it were that simple. The truth, of course, is that only someone much mightier than I knows the answer and it is not for me or any mere mortal to understand.

Certainly, few women have ever been more alike. And that's true even after I had promised myself in the year after Sally was gone what a mistake it would be to try to find someone like her. Then Bobbi entered my life and to this day I can't explain my good fortune.

Fun loving, aggressive, irreverent, witty, articulate and with an unbounded love and passion for all who were or are in need of help, neither Sally nor Bobbi knew how to say no, whether it was to a young mother with three tiny children going through the process of a painful divorce or to a woman newly diagnosed with breast cancer who sees her life crumbling out of control. Call Sally. Call Bobbi.

And both were filled with a fighting spirit that never knew the meaning of the word defeat.

Sally and I played tennis every Sunday and every other time we could. I had devised a system of slightly resizing the court on her side of the net so that our talents (such as they were) were evenly balanced. Every point--and every match--were fiercely competitive, and Sally hated to lose.

One Saturday night we had gone to a party and the beer flowed freely. When we stumbled onto the court the next day the temperature was in the mid 90s, with the humidity close behind. Not playing was *not* an option.

Somehow, probably because Sally felt even worse than I did, I droopily won the first two sets and went ahead 5-1 in the third. One more game, I told myself, and we could go home and try to find something to ease the throbbing in the head.

I served and Sally's return was weak. I lobbed the ball back across the net and stumbled forward for the kill. But I had made my shot too good. Sally came running up to it and from no more than 10 feet away took a vicious two-handed swing. I heard her racquet hit the ball and saw the ball coming straight at my eyes.

I fell to the court and looked back just in time to see the ball land inside the baseline and then slam up against the fence. I rolled over on my back on the blistering concrete surface and looked up to see Sally clenching the top of the net and glaring down at me. It was the second time I had seen fire coming from her dark eyes and she wasn't smiling.

"Get up," she screamed. "I've taken all of this crap I'm going to take. Now you get your ass back over there and we're going to play some real tennis."

I dragged myself to my feet and went back and served again. And the match went on. And on. And on for nearly another hour. Finally it was over and the score was 7-5 in my favor. But I knew who had really won.

Bobbi played with the same vigor, intensity and fortitude. After her mastectomy in 1986 she was told that she would have to undergo the experience of debilitating weekly chemotherapy.

Bobbi chose to do it through the heat of a Jacksonville summer and continued to play tennis weekly. How she did it I still don't know. Sometimes I could hardly bear to be on the court in the middle of the day myself -- and I was in reasonably good condition in those days.

But Bobbi never wavered. And she never complained. Sometimes I wondered if it was good for her physically. But mentally she proved that she could meet the challenge.

Conquering the employment hurdle was far different. One employer closed its Jacksonville office -- literally chained the door -- rather than continue in operation while having to provide medical coverage for a cancer "victim" (the employer's word--definitely not Bobbi's).

Bobbi fared no better with a well known cancer organization that seemed ready to hire her for an important position in its local operation until it found out. . . "Bobbi had cancer!"

Evidently it was OK to raise money for cancer research and preach the gospel of regular checkups for early detection and do all of the other good things. But hire someone who actually had cancer in a high profile position in its office? And provide for her continuing treatment and follow-up examinations? And what if she had a recurrence? How would *that* look?

Bobbi solved the problem by going to work for Florida Community College at Jacksonville, whose more tolerant and reasonable hiring policies were written by the State of Florida. Today she is with the Women's Center of Jacksonville and, of course, much has changed for the better over the last decade and a half.

Today, if someone develops cancer while employed, they are protected by the Americans with Disabilities Act and can be assured of keeping their jobs and benefits. Despite that, there are still unscrupulous employers who try to tell women with breast cancer that they're doing them a favor by "letting them go" so that they'll be eligible for disability or unemployment while recuperating. When Bobbi hears that, she goes ballistic, knowing full well what's behind this supposed kindness.

Cancer survivors today may have a better chance of getting a job after diagnosis, but there still is a long way to go. There are many ways to keep from hiring someone who is honest about having cancer. All an employer really has to say is, "We found someone more qualified." Women very often stay in a job they're unhappy with, or even stay in a marriage that's falling apart, just to keep those all important benefits. No one who's had cancer can ever afford to be without insurance. Bobbi knows. She's been there!

17

Bobbi's Story...

"Beam Me Up, Scotty"

We looked at all the options for treating my new cancer and decided that nuclear medicine was the best option. So we headed back to Tampa to be in the capable hands of Dr. Klotch.

It was January 2000 and I began the new millennium by spending a week in isolation while being treated for metastatic thyroid cancer. Just me, a bed, a television set, a telephone and three hazardous waste containers.

I remember arriving at the hospital not having a clue of exactly what being in isolation entailed. To this day I'm not sure if it was real or simply a bad dream.

I went through the usual reams of paperwork necessary to be admitted to the Moffitt Cancer Center in Tampa and then I was on my own. It didn't make any sense for Jerry to be in Tampa with me since I would not be allowed to have any visitors during my period of isolation. I was warned ahead of time that anything I brought into isolation with me would either have to be thrown away or remain there for 90 days "in quarantine" to make sure it was free of radioactivity before they let me take it home. It was a difficult time. I couldn't imagine being in the hospital and not having Jerry, my sister Adrienne or my mother with me. I don't think I was fearful but I certainly was perplexed.

At least I knew what caused this cancer. When I was a child between the age of one and two, I was treated with radiation for a thymus gland problem. It wasn't until I was in my teens that we learned that young children treated with radiation had a 38 percent higher risk of getting thyroid cancer. Thank heavens they don't use that form of treatment anymore. If it had been detected earlier and had not spread, I would have been home free. But now they were going to use a form of radiation to "cure" the cancer that was caused by radiation in the first place. No wonder I was perplexed.

After I went through several body scans that would be used for before and after treatment comparisons, I was taken up to my room and "settled in." What an eerie feeling.

The red hazardous waste containers were huge and stood right in front of my bed. Since I was going to be treated with radioactivity, I had to throw all paper plates and plastic utensils away after each meal. I learned that the radioactivity was secreted through my bodily fluids so I also had to throw my underwear away each day. It was actually a good opportunity to get rid of all of the old underwear my mother always warned me against wearing in case I was in an accident.

Then two nuclear medicine technicians wheeled a steel container into my room. It looked like a mini bank vault. They asked if I was ready. Could anyone ever be ready for a scenario as weird as that? One of the technicians took a small vial out of the "vault" with gloved hands, handed it to me and said, "Drink up. We'll see you in a week." Then they left. Jerry's cousin Phyllis Fabara and her husband Leslie had sent me a bunch of paperback books and a little Beanie Baby silver tiger named "Plata," which means silver in Spanish. Plata became my link to the outside world. It's a good thing no one could hear my conversations with Plata or I would have never been let out of isolation.

There was a steel shield around my bed and my meals were brought in by someone covered from head to toe in protective gear. I remember having a paper thermometer and paper blood pressure cuff. No one wanted to be in there with me any longer than a minute. They weren't a danger to me. I was a danger to them. I was radioactive from the isotopes being used to kill any leftover cancerous cells in my body.

I thought I could use the time to rest and catch up on some much needed sleep. But I found it impossible to sleep. It wasn't that I felt sick. I didn't really feel anything. But I was used to working 40 plus hours a week and running support groups at night and catching up on housework and yard work on weekends. I was like a well-oiled machine that had suddenly ground to a halt. I rarely have a chance to watch television, but while I was in isolation I read during the day and watched television all night. I simply couldn't sleep and the weird environment didn't help. I had thought about bringing my laptop computer with me so that I could write about my experiences, but it, too, would have been quarantined for 90 days.

The one week felt like a lifetime. I lived for my daily phone calls from Jerry, my sister Adrienne and my Bosom Buddies. The hardest thing of all was being separated from my great support system. I saved all the "love notes" I received during that time and will never part with them. Phone calls from my friend Paula Thompson picked my spirits up. She kept me laughing and that's just what I needed.

This period of time gave me a great opportunity to think about my life and my work in cancer survivorship. I focused inwardly and wondered if I was really making a difference. Helping other women who were just starting out on their cancer journey had become my life. So many people told me to "put it behind me. Get on with life." At the end of my time in isolation with nothing to do but think and reflect about the wondrous people I had met since 1986, survivors and caregivers alike, I knew with every fiber of my being that this was exactly what I wanted to be doing with my life. As long as there were women still being diagnosed with breast cancer, I wanted to be there for them.

At the end of the week, two more nuclear medicine technicians came into my room with a Geiger counter of sorts. If the radioactivity in my body measured under "30 rads," an acronym for radiation-absorbed dose, I could leave. Thank heavens I met the test. I was going home.

As I left the isolation room, I noticed there were two sets of doors between my room and the hospital corridor. There were huge caution signs posted and yellow tape all around the frame of my room. As I stepped into the corridor everyone eyed me as if I were "typhoid Mary." So I just strolled on by and said, "Beam me up, Scotty. Just think. I'll never need another Halloween costume. I already glow in the dark."

That wasn't really the end of it. For the next two weeks I couldn't be around any small children. I couldn't sit next to my husband in the van. I had to ride in the back. I couldn't even sleep in the same room with him and I had to keep my personal laundry and the dishes I used apart from the rest of the household. I couldn't wait for the two additional weeks to end. I was raring to go back to work and a normal lifestyle. I was in remission again and I hoped it was for life this time.

All of this turmoil was going on while I was in the process of moving Bosom Buddies from the community college, where it had been housed since 1988, to the Women's Center of Jacksonville. I was on the brink of making my dream of running Bosom Buddies on a full-time basis come true. When I knew I was going to retire from the college, I began to look into a variety of nonprofit agencies in Jacksonville to see which one would be a good fit for Bosom Buddies.

It must have been divine guidance that put me together with the Women's Center. Its mission is to support and empower women by nurturing mind, body and spirit and by advocating for the dignity and respect of all women.

Bosom Buddies' mission is to inform, educate and provide heart-to-heart emotional support to those diagnosed with breast cancer; to encourage recognition of the need for early detection; to teach women to advocate their needs while empowering them with the knowledge that will enable them to become full partners in making decisions about essential health care. What a perfect fit!

Finally the day came when I was sitting in my college office surrounded by 12 years in the life of Bosom Buddies, all boxed up and me too weak to lift a single box. Peggy Ryan-Smith, one of my Bosom Buddies and the wife of an officer at Jacksonville Naval Air Station, came to my rescue. She turned up with a crew of friends and nurses from the Naval Hospital and said, "You just sit there. We'll do the moving." And move they did. Box after box after box, with the help of Bettina Cross, my student assistant. When our caravan of cars and vans arrived at the Women's Center we all wondered how it would all fit in a quarter of the space I had before. I remembered what my mother always said, "Where there's love, there's room," and with all the love pouring out from from these women we pushed, shoved and stacked boxes until there wasn't enough room for a match stick.

I had found a second home for Bosom Buddies. But more than that, I found myself surrounded by the most dynamic, caring women I'd ever had the privilege of working with, most of them 15 to 35 years younger than I was. Women like Shirley Webb, our executive director and founder of the first shelter for battered women in Jacksonville; Milanie Hatfield, queen of community education; Elizabeth Fattorusso, who shored up whatever department needed help with her myriad of talents while raising her son as a single mom; Maura Driscoll, an intern who we were smart enough to keep; our Rape Recovery Team members, Kim Kelly, Bina Patel, Heather Buckman and Michelle Meyers, on duty 24/7 aiding victims of sexual assault, and our beloved Audrey Dearborn, who was responsible for the support program for women with HIV AIDS.

I knew from the first moment that the only way they'd get me to leave the Women's Center would be feet first . . . and then I'd probably still come back to haunt them. I knew at last that Bosom Buddies had finally come home. What was important to me was that if the day ever comes when I'm either unable to work or I really decide to retire, the mission and the work of Bosom Buddies will go on. I am awed by the caliber of the young women around me and know full well that they have the love and ability to keep Bosom Buddies on the right track.

It was time to take my show on the road for life.

18

Jerry's Story...

Breast Cancer: Past, Present and Future

It always hurts me to see little pieces of Bobbi's heart chipped away when someone in Bosom Buddies runs out of time. I share her frustration in the ups and downs of breast cancer detection and treatment and I'm still appalled that more than 40,000 women are losing their lives every year.

It's like taking 10 giant steps forward and five giant steps backward. I never cease to marvel at how women live on this seesaw called survivorship. For many years, the emphasis was on early detection through breast self-examination and mammography. Now that's all questionable. Some new research shows that there is very little difference in the length of survival between women who follow the program for early detection and those who don't. How can that possibly be? How long can these women wait for a cure?

Without organizations like Bosom Buddies, how would newly diagnosed women determine the best road to survivorship? The greatest thing about support groups is that the "veterans" take the "rookies" under their wing, convincing them there's good, productive life after cancer. There's nothing better than getting information straight from someone who's been there herself. I only wish the spouses or significant others in these women's lives felt that way about getting support for themselves. It doesn't come easy for men.

Every woman who's been diagnosed can remember the exact moment they were told they had breast cancer. The "D" day which stands for diagnosis. But no one ever says, "Today you're cured."

All of which leads me to a survey I did in 1999 of my graduate school class in journalism. We were all together -- 68 of us -- at Columbia University in New York City in 1956-57. After we graduated most of the class members went on to careers in journalism or closely allied endeavors that gave them a ringside seat on history as it unfolded in the last 42 years of the 20th Century.

One went on to become executive editor of *TIME* magazine. Another became *TIME's* White House correspondent. One became the producer of Walter Cronkite's nightly news broadcast on television. One became publisher of Canada's largest newspaper. Others went on to key positions with major wire services and TV networks and newspapers in New York, Rome, Bonn, Los Angeles, Miami, Washington, Salt Lake City, Louisville, Omaha, Anchorage, Saigon, Tokyo and wherever the news of the world was happening. One even spent Christmas in Nome, Alaska, just to see what it was like. Several wrote books. Others became professors of journalism and public relations and history and some went into industry and one spent several years in the aerospace program. One even entered politics. She did pretty well, too and became the first woman governor of Vermont, won re-election, and then became our ambassador to Switzerland. Her name is Madeleine May Kunin.

None of this is intended to dazzle anyone but rather to establish the class members as people who have been, and in many cases still are, close to what's going on in the world. Just before we graduated in 1957 I was elected permanent class secretary and asked to do an annual newsletter of where the class members were and what they were doing. I thought that after a year or two interest would wane and my assignment would quietly be forgotten. I was wrong. The job goes on and I still put out a newsletter each December.

As we approached the new millennium in late 1999 I decided it would be fun to poll members of the class on what they thought were the top three news stories or news developments in the 42 years since we had graduated. At the top of the list, as it turned out, was the breakup of the Soviet Union, the end of the Cold War and the reunification of Germany. In second place were mankind's triumphs in space, led by the landing of astronauts on the moon. In third place was microminiaturization, combined with the development of the computer and the internet.

That was half the survey, the easy part. The other half was for each class member to look into the future for the same length of time and rank the top three news stories or news developments expected to occur between 2000 and 2042.

The top choice: A cure for cancer!

This, they predicted, will be the most newsworthy development over the next 42 or 43 years. Bigger than major societal changes in the way we live, due to the aging of the American population and the impact of today's minorities becoming tomorrow's majorities (and vice versa), which ranked second. Bigger than new scientific and technological breakthroughs, and especially finding a replacement for fossil fuels, which ranked third. Bigger than global disasters, manmade and natural, which ranked fourth.

No one predicted the cataclysmic events of September 11, 2001, but that hardly diminishes the considered opinion of so many in the class that a cure for cancer will be found. Most of them based their belief on advances in genetic engineering. Many of them also expressed the belief that rather than one miracle cure being found for all cancer, there will be a more gradual, but nonetheless certain, progression of cures for cancer in all of its many forms. And several class members also predicted a concurrent development of a means for cancer prevention.

Unless you're reading this in 2043 or later, who knows how accurate the prediction will be? But even as this is being written, hardly a day goes by when there is not at least one news story about another significant breakthrough in cancer research, detection and treatment. Can a cure (and prevention) be far behind?

If nothing else, it all adds up to one more reason for hope for the future.

19

Bobbi's Story...

"Get a Life." I'd Love One, Thank You!

I can't help it. The evil just comes bubbling out of me when people say things like, "You're so lucky. You had a 'good' cancer," when they talk about my having had metastatic thyroid cancer. Or, "You're cured, what more do you want?" when they talk about my advanced breast cancer. Especially since we know that's not really true where breast cancer is concerned. We don't have to define our lives by having had cancer, but it will always be a part of us. There's no getting away from that. Only someone who has never faced a life-threatening illness would say some of the insensitive things we're told as cancer survivors.

Over the last two decades, I seem to be spending more time at doctors' offices than I do spending time on more pleasant things, like working out, getting a manicure, visiting the grandchildren and many other relaxing things. Don't get me wrong. I'm not whining about this. I'm one of the lucky ones. I'm still here. It's just that it gets old. Ask any long-term survivor and they'll tell you the very same thing.

Let's face it. Cancer does affect your life forever. I'm not saying that's all bad either. But we have to deal with a new sense of normal. I'm not being flippant when I say, "Get a life. I'd love one thank you!" I just want to know who I am now. I'm not the same person I was B.C. (before cancer) – and maybe that's not all bad. I no longer feel corny when I tell my friends, family and Bosom Buddies, I love you, over and over again. And that's because I now realize how important it is to share your feelings with those you love. I also say "please" and "thank you" much more than I ever did before. I think having an uncertain future goes along with that. Yes, I cry when I see the American flag flying over war-torn areas. I cry when I see pictures of children diagnosed with cancer. I cry when beautiful music touches my soul and I cry when time runs out for a very dear friend. And I won't apologize for any of these abundant emotions. It means I'm alive and kicking and I feel the ups and downs of life. I guess that's the new me. That's part of being a cancer warrior.

I know what it's like to want to "stop and smell the roses." I not only want to smell them, I also want to play in the dirt and plant them. I have a sense of wanting to be around living things much more than I ever did before fighting cancer. Early on in our Bosom Buddies history, when we were located at Florida Community College in Jacksonville, we started a memorial garden. When one of our beloved buddies passed away, we shared a tree planting in her memory with her family. It was an incredible experience to see Coleen Choley's two young sons actually dig the hole and plant the tree for their mom. Over the years we watched it grow as the boys grew and realized how much that tree came to mean to all of us. It was a living symbol that lasted long after Coleen left on her heavenly journey, and that was important to all of us. Nearly two decades later, we're still planting memorial trees and it still makes us feel better as we watch the young tree grow upward toward the sun, as strong and beautiful as the person who left us on another journey.

One of the biggest changes is my life is my newfound spiritual sense. I guess it was always there under the surface and maybe it took a cancer journey to bring it out. I always objected to what I called "organized religion." Now I welcome it in my life. The formality of attending a service along with the rituals of worship have a much deeper meaning to me now. There's a sense of comfort that goes along with it that wasn't there before. I know prayer works and I work at prayer. I spend time each day thanking God for another day and I never fail to pray for my fellow survivors who need extra intervention. And I've seen a lot of miracles.

It was this newfound spiritual sense that brought the biggest change in my life. Jerry's religion has always been an integral part of his life and the life of his children. I never had children of my own and when our grandchildren Anna Carr and Cole came along, I wanted to be close to them in every way. When they were baptized and I found myself on the outside looking in, I began to think what it would mean for all of us to be able to worship together. I mentioned that to Jerry one day and he suggested I go to church with him on Sunday. When I walked up to the entrance to San Jose Episcopal Church, I was greeted with a welcoming smile and a hug from Betsy Kemp, who was one of the greeters that day. Before I knew what was happening, I became a member of the choir, singing to the glory of the Lord. As I sang and prayed, I realized that I could be a part of this without ever really losing my Jewish roots. No one else thought less of me because I wasn't an Episcopalian. I jokingly said that I had created my own special religion and that I was an "Episcayiddle." I meant that in the most loving sense. I felt I had the best of both worlds. Singing in the choir under the direction of Bill Peters was a thrill for me. Music was finally back in my life and I couldn't wait to get to church on Sunday and sing. No matter how difficult the week was, I always left after service feeling good and positive about life.

As time went on and I became more involved in various ministries of the church, I began to feel a sense of peace and belonging. I came to the difficult decision that I wanted to become an Episcopalian in the true sense of the word. I spent a long time thinking about what I should do.

Then, after singing one night before Thanksgiving, I felt that I had come to a fork in the road of my life and decided to go forward with plans to become a full-fledged member of the church. I've never regretted that decision nor will I ever abandon my Jewish origin. I am proud of my heritage and will never deny it. Joining the church added another wonderful dimension to my life and to my marriage. Jerry and I could now worship together.

20

Jerry's Story . . .

"The Good News of Survival"

I'm sure I'd heard the expression before but it never quite struck me the way it did on this particular Sunday morning.

The Rev. Larry Wilkes was assistant rector at San Jose Episcopal Church in Jacksonville. He was delivering a sermon on a subject with a different focus than cancer when he started talking about the good news of survival.

I remember sitting straight up in the pew. That's it, I thought. The Good News of Survival. That's really what Bobbi and I are talking about when we share our stories with other cancer survivors and caregivers in Springfield, Massachusetts, and Atlanta, Georgia, and Victoria, British Columbia, and dozens of other cities across the United States and Canada.

The Good News of Survival. The wonderful people you meet. The friends you make. The unforgettable experiences. And the joy of new hope as the sun rises each day to begin its journey across the heavens.

We all know that cancer has its tears, and its feelings of loneliness, despair and hopelessness. But it also possesses its moments of joy and thoughtfulness even though it may sometimes take years to appreciate them in their fullness.

I'll never forget how Louise Carlucci walked into my life as I sat outside the operating suite where Sally's first surgery was getting ready to take place. I sat there shivering in fear when Louise walked into the almost empty waiting room shortly after 6 o'clock that morning. I knew who she was because our firm had helped her husband, Joe Carlucci, win election to the Florida Senate. For a moment I wondered why Louise was there and I quickly decided that she must also know someone scheduled for surgery that morning.

But she came directly over to where I was sitting and sat down beside me, and when I looked at her she said very softly, "I heard about Sally's surgery and I was afraid you might be here all by yourself."

A few minutes later A. C. Soud walked in and came over to join us. A. C. was a local attorney who had served as treasurer of Joe Carlucci's political campaign. After he sat down he said, "I wonder if we could bow our heads in prayer?"

Hours later Louise and A.C. were still there for me to lean on when the surgeon emerged from the operating room and told me that a serious recurrence of Sally's ovarian cancer had been detected.

A. C. never did practice law that morning. A few years later we helped him become elected as a circuit judge, a position he still serves with dignity and distinction. But I'll always remember him and Louise most for those moments we shared together with our heads bowed in prayer in the chill of that surgical waiting room.

There are many others I'll never forget, like David Harrell, and his unlimited offer of financial support. And Father John Riley, who guided me through Sally's illness and the glory of her funeral and then, a few years later, donned a Jewish yarmulke to marry Bobbi and me in the study of his Episcopal Church. Father John is pretty much retired today but we still run into each other at the dry cleaners and other places and his first word of greeting is always a hearty, "Shalom!"

And there was Louise Grange, the wife of Gifford Grange, who also was mentioned earlier in the book for preserving my sanity (and perhaps my life) on the night before Sally's funeral. Louise and several other friends made sure there was always ample food in the house for the steady flow of family members and friends who came by every day to visit Sally and comfort her.

You never forget people like that, or the neighbors who lived nearby on Woodward Avenue in Jacksonville.

Sally's diagnosis touched off an almost daily schedule of hospital treatment, with each appointment taking several hours. But the public relations firm I owned provided our only means of financial support and I needed to spend as much time as possible in the office each day. I called a very prominent cancer organization to see if some means of transportation and assistance could be arranged and was told very curtly, "We don't do that sort of thing."

Then the women in the neighborhood learned of our predicament. And Sally never missed an appointment.

One of our firm's clients was B. J. Strickland, who owned several of Jacksonville's most popular restaurants. He also was known for throwing some of the city's most lavish parties. One day as we were wrapping up a meeting together he asked how Sally was doing. I tried to be upbeat but I guess the look on my face gave me away and B. J. detected that Sally's condition was growing more serious by the day.

"I have an idea," B.J. said. "Why don't you let us have a party for Sally? Invite all of her friends. We'll provide everything."

"B. J.," I replied, "that's very kind but I don't think Sally is strong enough to spend three or four hours at the Town House standing on her feet and greeting everyone, as much as she might want to."

"Then let's forget the Town House," B.J. said. "What if we catered it at your house? We'll also provide the servers and clean up afterward."

And that's what he did. It was one of those wonderful parties where everyone came. And stayed. Sally loved people and this was the night everyone showed how they felt about Sally.

It was well after midnight when B.J.'s people had cleaned up everything and the last guests were gone. Sally and I were alone and I went over to the chair where she had spent the evening greeting her friends. Her face was covered with tears of joy. I had never seen her look so happy or so peaceful. B.J.'s party was a success -- and two weeks later Sally was gone.

Who could ever forget B.J. Strickland? Or Sally's doctor, Irvin Schneider? What made Irvin Schneider so different wasn't his medical acumen, which I never had reason to question. What made him unforgettable was his kindness and understanding. Like the times he reminded me, "Jerry, my home telephone number is in the phone book. I want you to use it and call me at home at any time you want. And I don't care if it's on weekends or at 2 o'clock in the morning. You call me when you need me." I wonder how many other doctors say that to their patients and their caregivers?

And then there was my son J.R. He attended Episcopal High School in Jacksonville and was a starter on the basketball team. On the night of Sally's funeral, Episcopal had a game scheduled and I told J.R. to go ahead and play. More than that, I told him I'd bring Grandpa Jerry (my father) with me and we'd see the game together. Dad thought that was a wonderful idea. It would relieve our sadness and, since he lived in Arkansas, it would give him a chance to see J.R. play.

The Episcopal gym at the time was quite small. We arrived early enough to take a couple of seats directly under the basket at one end of the court, no more than six feet from the playing area itself.

A short time later, as the team was leaving the floor after its pre-game warm-up, J.R. came over to where Dad and I were sitting. He bent over in front of us and looked straight into my eyes and said quietly but firmly, "Dad, I just want you to know that this game's for you." Then he got up and ran and joined his teammates.

To be truthful, Episcopal did not really have all that great a team, but on this particular night the team played well and the lead seemed to change with every basket scored. Finally, with time running out and only seconds remaining on the clock, Episcopal trailed by one.

What happened next I still find hard to believe. While trying to get off one final shot that would put the lead -- and the game itself -- back in Episcopal's favor, J.R. was fouled.

There were three seconds left to play as J.R. moved to the foul line at our end of the court for the first of his two free throws.

J.R. stood at the foul line and bounced the ball once. Then twice. Then, for one split second, without turning his head, he took his eyes off the basket and glanced over at me as if to reaffirm his promise. Then he arced the ball toward the basket. It swished through the net and the game was tied. J.R. got the ball back and shot again. And again the shot was good. Episcopal led by one and three seconds later the game was over.

I leaped up and dashed onto the court and threw my arms around J.R. And this time the tears of joy were on my face.

Many years later, after we had helped relocate Dad to Jacksonville, he and I were enjoying a drink together before dinner when he asked, "Do you still remember the night of Sally's funeral when you and I went to see J.R.'s basketball game and how J.R. came over before the game and said that he was dedicating the game to you? And then how he made those two shots in the last few seconds that won the game?"

"Dad," I said, "I'll never forget it."

"Neither will I," he smiled. Dad had just turned 99 years old.

Memories like these are the good news of survival. . . and survivorship. If there's a moral to all of this it's not only to know that there are tears of joy in being a cancer survivor and caregiver but also to remember that the kindness and thoughtfulness you share with others are what help produce those tears of joy.

21

Bobbi's Story

"Heroes Are Everywhere"

When I was diagnosed in 1986, women with Stage IV metastatic breast cancer had only a small chance of surviving. Now, I see many of my Bosom Buddies living good productive lives with advanced breast cancer. Yes, they may be on treatment for the rest of their lives, but at least they're still here to talk about it. I salute their courage and determination. There's a world of heroes out there and I have the privilege of calling many of them "beloved friends."

Two of my very special heroes are Barbara Whalen and Marj Zaros. Diagnosed with Stage IV metastatic breast cancer from the very beginning, these warrior women let nothing stand in their way. They live life to the fullest, even though they are constantly on one treatment protocol after another. They don't whine over their situation. Instead, they ask "What else is out there that I haven't tried?"

My heart swells with pride as I watch these women fight the good fight. They won't take no for an answer when the doctor says there's really nothing else left to try. Marj has traveled from coast to coast, seeking out every new clinical trial available to her. Her zest for life, and that of Barbara, is unsinkable and their faith in a higher power is stronger than the rock of Gibraltar.

Barbara, Marj and many others inspired me to ask the question, "What are the best things about being a breast cancer survivor?" Many of the answers I received were things I experienced myself and were not surprising. Others brought tears to my eyes. Here are some of the things they had to say:

Jane Kowalski

"Many of the things I've learned while surviving cancer myself I've been able to turn around and use in my job as a practicing nurse. Like being able to say to a patient who's going through treatment, 'I know just how you feel.' Or being able to take my Cancer Survivors Cookbook along so that the Home Health Aides can make the best food possible. And being able to share those little tried and true tips that got me through cancer. Or laughing with my patients about the awful side effects of treatment, something you wouldn't normally be able to even talk about. Or being able to say with all sincerity how important each day is and how grateful you are just to wake up in the morning. And knowing how to style a patient's wig and make her look like a million dollars with scarves and makeup. And understanding the importance of doing something today if that is what your patient wants because tomorrow may be too late. And lastly, to listen to your inner voice. I was given a letter by one of my patients about how she wanted to die. My inner voice told me the most important thing to do that evening was to give it to her daughters and tell them to read it, right away. My patient died several hours later in exactly the way she wanted.

"Survivorship brings a bond and a trust between us -- a love and relationship that can never be eroded. I feel connected to a spiritual world and taken care of by my guardian angels. In a way I feel a wholeness. I feel blessed to join my sisters in this world of survivorship, a companionship so beautiful, so warm, so clear and so honest. I feel lucky. Live in hope, pray in faith, believe in miracles. We are miracles!"

Peg Chassman

"Knowing that people care and want to help. That's what counted to me. It didn't matter if I knew the people or not. A lot of people from all over the world reached out to me. It made me realize that it was a good opportunity for me to reach out to other women who also have been diagnosed with breast cancer or are having a potential problem with a mammogram or ultrasound and are scared stiff. I will go to appointments with them or just be there for them. I realize how important it is to be in a support group. I've gained a lot of new friends through Bosom Buddies and value our camaraderie. Most of all, this has all made me see what I always knew, what a great husband I have. He has gone through this journey with me and is always at my side."

Pamela Murphy

"Since I was 12 I have been taking care of my mother, which is a real role reversal. She is now in her late '70s and the role is still the same. I used to carry a great deal of anger in my heart because I never had a typical mother/daughter relationship. My mother has never been lacking in anything from me, but I often felt empty. All of that anger is gone now and there is pure joy and love in my heart. I have found acceptance and peace in the relationship. I now enjoy each moment we have. We laugh a lot more and to this day she does not know about my own illness."

Molly McRae

"Three positive things that come to mind right away are that a cancer diagnosis causes you to get your priorities in order, if they're not already; that life and its blessings really do seem a little sweeter, and that less is taken for granted and even the ordinary is appreciated."

Lori Covell

"I have found out how much I am loved by my family. I've always known it, but never felt it so strongly until my diagnosis. Now I feel even deeper in love with my husband. I don't want to take him for granted for even a minute. I've gained some really wonderful friends that I never would have known if I hadn't been diagnosed with cancer. It's changed my outlook on life from 'a glass half empty' to 'a glass half full.'"

Carolyn Disher-Ryan

"Meeting and making new friends, especially those who are also survivors and understand what's going on. That's so important. And so is getting closer to God, my husband and my children. And being able to talk about death, which I would never have done with the family. And being able to decide what is important in my life and what's not important.

"I remember going to my first Bosom Buddies meeting in 1995 and just hearing everyone talk. When it was my turn, I could only cry. Everyone said just the right things to me at the right time. That really helped and still continues to help me with the positive attitude everyone has."

Cecilia Kress

"I try to enjoy life and focus on its positive aspects. I've become more spiritual than before. I don't get upset when things go wrong. We need to enjoy ourselves and others."

Connie Hildebrand

"When I hear others saying they had a bad day, I think to myself that there is no such thing as a bad day as long as I'm alive and able to wake up and have another day tomorrow. There's no such thing as a bad hair day. I will take hair anyway I can get it!

Love comes to us in ways we are not expecting. Sometimes it's the soft nuzzle of a cold kitty nose or a dog's loving gaze when he wants to be petted. And most of all, there really is a God and he is paying attention."

Denise Jones

"I have a renewed faith in God and pray for others while often forgetting to pray for myself. I've made more friends than I could ever have imagined from Bosom Buddies. I learned how to take my own heath care into my hands, rather than just trusting doctors. All my life I did whatever a doctor told me to do, but I've learned the importance of self-education and to question my treatment path.

"I'm amazed at how willing people are to help me when I tell them I have breast cancer. Strangers have hugged me and told me they will pray for me and given me gifts. It is just unbelievable. Before, I felt that most people could care less about others. I definitely learned who was a true friend. Neighbors and friends have called and volunteered to drive me to my chemo or radiation treatments and made me promise to call them if I needed help.

"One neighbor brought me a wig and scarves from a friend of hers who had breast cancer. Another printed out literature about breast cancer. Others sent family members to help fix my house when they learned I had a problem. I have learned that the most important thing is to live each day to the fullest and the other things will take care of themselves. I live for today, don't think about what I should have done, and look forward to tomorrow."

Linda Cornelio

"Having had breast cancer awakened a desire in me to help myself and others by finding little known information to aid in survival. I have always loved to read and that has served me well. In addition, God blessed me with a good mind which enables me not only to seek out the information, but also to understand it and remember it. Being able to help other women through my research and knowledge has brought me great pleasure. It has also created an instant bond with other survivors when we see each other's pink ribbons."

Mary Graves

"I count every year as precious these days. I want everyone to know that I am 57 years ALIVE! I'm glad that cancer brought so many new friends into my life. Everything is more -- joys are more joyful, peace is more peaceful, family and friends are more precious, trees are more green, and even heaven is more desirable. Everything is more, except problems. They seem smaller and less significant.

"Life is seen in its essence. Pouring oneself out for others in Jesus' name is our purpose. Life is also seen in its transcendence. God is ever present, and his presence is so precious.

"Cancer teaches many lessons about living. These lessons can be meaningfully shared with others who are just beginning their walk"

You can see by these comments from some of my Bosom Buddies why these women mean so much to me. They've been able to take a devastating experience and see something good come out of it. As longtime survivor Susan Matsuko Shinagawa says in the title of the inspiring song she wrote, "Heroes Are Everywhere."

22

Jerry's Story

"On the Road for Life"

Bobbi had already been journeying around the country and speaking about cancer survivorship for many years when I joined her in 1998. I really wasn't sure that anyone would be interested in what I had to say about cancer survivorship. I have never considered myself an "expert" on the subject (and still don't) and all I could really do was relate my personal experiences in caring for Sally and Bobbi.

Much to my surprise, I found that was enough, especially when I broadened my experiences and words of encouragement to include both caregivers and survivors.

Now that I've spent many years "On the Road for Life" with Bobbi, I can truly say that joining her was perhaps the most enjoyable, and meaningful, decision I've ever made. We travel throughout the United States and Canada, speaking in cities, and to audiences, large and small.

Bobbi and I often say that if we reach just one or two people in each audience and inspire them with new hope and a renewed sense of purpose in their life after cancer, then we have done our job. Of course, we hope that we reach a whole lot more than just one or two.

For reasons we've never figured out, almost all of our speaking engagements have been in a wide arc stretching from South Florida to the Pacific Northwest, including Vancouver and Victoria, British Columbia. We've been to much of the Rocky Mountain area, the Midwest, the South and the East, but the closest we've ever been to the Pacific Southwest is Modesto, California, some 80 miles east of Sacramento.

We've been to the Chicago area twice and Atlanta three times, and we've been to Boise, Salt Lake City, Oklahoma City, Miami and many places you've probably never heard of.

Like Plentywood, Montana. Get a magnifying glass and a map and look closely in the extreme northeastern corner of the state. There, on the High Plains, about 120 miles south of Regina, Saskatchewan, and 100 miles northwest of Williston, North Dakota, is Plentywood. Population 2,061. We spoke there in conjunction with another engagement in Glasgow, Montana, population 3,253.

We spoke in Plentywood on a Saturday night and by the time we had wrapped things up it was nearly 9 o'clock. Since we had to speak the next day in Glasgow, our sponsors thought it best to drive us right back to Glasgow, a mere 160 miles away. On the entire three-hour trip, if I remember correctly, we passed exactly 11 moving vehicles—and 25 deer.

But the emptiness of northeastern Montana is part of its fascination and the few people who live there . . . well consider this. On the night we arrived in Glasgow, after we had registered for our motel room, the clerk at the desk handed us a second set of keys.

"These are for the green Buick parked out front," he said. "The people who invited you thought you might enjoy taking a drive around the area after you have breakfast tomorrow morning." Where else would that happen?

When we were in Youngstown, Ohio, our hosts took us out for a sumptuous dinner one night and then one of them drove us back to our motel. On the way, she asked, "Would you people like some ice cream? There's a great little place just ahead."

So she pulled in and we stood outside in the parking lot enjoying the best ice cream sundaes Bobbi and I have ever tasted. Little things like that may not seem like much, but they have a special meaning when you're 800 miles from home.

Then there were the people at the Potlatch Corporation who wanted us to speak to the paper mill workers at their plant in Brainerd, Minnesota. Bobbi and I weren't sure we were really the speakers they wanted, since much of Bobbi's presentation is aimed at breast cancer survivors and the audience would consist almost solely of men. But Potlatch was insistent, so Bobbi and I went to Brainerd and spoke to what we both now agree were three of the most attentive audiences we've ever faced.

In one afternoon, we did three one-hour presentations, each one packed with at least a hundred Paul Bunyan-size mill workers, many of whom could not find a seat and had to stand or sit on the concrete floor. After each presentation there was time for us to meet the workers and we were bombarded with some of the most intelligent and insightful questions we've ever been asked, on subjects ranging from the mind-body connection to guided imagery and the importance of a healthy lifestyle.

We were so pressed for time that for lunch, our host for the day had to call out and have some pizzas delivered. That was more than enough. For the chance to talk with those workers, Bobbi and I would have gone hungry.

And sometimes we make long-time friends, like Linda Brown with the Roger Maris Cancer Center in Fargo, North Dakota, who invited us to speak in 2002 and has been an e-mail friend ever since – along with her cats Henry and Louise.

Funny things happen, too, like the time we were checking our bags in Boise, Idaho, for the return flight to Jacksonville. We were the only ones checking in at the time and for some reason the agent at the check-in counter decided we needed to have our bags opened and inspected. With that he called over a security officer who looked at me and asked, "Which bag would you like me to inspect, sir?"

I thought he was kidding but I quickly decided that if I told him the bag on the left, he'd check the one on the right – or vice versa. We certainly had nothing to hide so I pointed to the bag on the left. Believe it or not, that's the one he opened. Then, after shuffling through our dirty clothes, he said, "Thank you very much, sir. Have a nice flight." You figure it out.

Every trip is a great experience (well, almost every one) and we've met some absolutely wonderful people. In all of our travels, we've only had one bad experience and even there we became friends with a cancer survivor who still sends us an occasional e-mail.

In turn, Bobbi and I have gained a reputation, which I hope we deserve, of being two of the most accommodating speakers who do this sort of thing. We simply believe, that when someone is nice enough to invite us to speak we should do it all, including media interviews, special presentations, guest appearances and anything else we're asked to do. Bobbi and I are always amazed when we're told about other speakers who demand to be picked up at the airport in a chauffer-driven limousine, or that they will only stay at a four or five-star hotel, or that their bed sheets be a certain color (and we're not exaggerating).

We're also fortunate to have a wonderful agent named Mike Dowling, who makes most of the initial contacts for our speaking engagements. Mike is both caring and conscientious, and Bobbi and I try to fulfill the impression that Mike creates when he books engagements for us.

That's what it's like – being "On the Road for Life."

23

Bobbi's Story...

The Next Bend in the Road

When I began my cancer journey in 1986, I had no idea what was in store for me. I think now how presumptuous it was for me to think of starting a support group for women like myself. What did I know about breast cancer? Not very much. I certainly never imagined that I would be involved in the survivorship movement on a national level. I felt very strongly that medical coverage for everyone should be a right, not a privilege, and that's basically why I became involved with the Intercultural Cancer Council (ICC) after my term on the board of directors of the NCCS.

The ICC is the nation's largest multicultural and multidisciplinary organization that promotes policies, programs, partnerships and research to address the unequal burden of cancer among ethnic and racial minorities and the medically underserved of all races. My many years on its board of governors has taught me that access to health insurance usually means if you can afford it, you can get it. That's a whole different meaning than coverage for everyone, regardless of your ability to pay for the care.

The ICC was co-founded by Lovell Jones, Ph.D., director of the Center for Research on Minority Health at the University of Texas MD Anderson Cancer Center, and Armin Weinberg, Ph.D., director of the Chronic Disease Prevention and Control Research Center at Baylor College of Medicine. The glue that holds the ICC together is the tireless Pamela Jackson, director of Outreach Programs and the ICC National Network, along with Jay Silver, its executive director. This organization has done more to call attention to the disparities that exist in health care than any other organization and this inspired me to fight for the rights of cancer survivors on a whole different level. While finding a cure for cancer is of vital importance, leveling the field so that everyone has the same access to quality cancer care and research is of equal importance. One of my greatest pleasures was creating the ICC's slogan, "Speaking With One Voice." And we really mean that.

I see advances being made every day in research that hopefully will give us the answer to why the mortality rate for African American women with breast cancer is so much greater than the mortality rate for Caucasian women when the incidence of breast cancer in African American women is considerably less. This is not just a socioeconomic problem. It's a problem of understanding different cultures and respecting the beliefs that may keep certain women from seeking help when a problem with their health arises.

I'm proud to serve with people like Susan Matsuko Shinagawa, past chair of the ICC, who despite her own difficulties with recurrent breast cancer, has made the world a better place for Asian Americans with cancer. My life has been tremendously enriched by her friendship.

I have worked side-by-side with fellow survivors Jim Williams, Venus Gínes, Catherine Logan Carrillo, Ivis Febus-Sampayo and Annie Mary Johnson, whose command of the English language, perfectly articulated, makes everyone stand up and take notice.

What I know best as a cancer survivor, and one who works with cancer communities around the country, is that the incidence and survival rates within cultural groups provide a uniform way of portraying the cancer problem from an ethnic perspective. From these statistics, health care practitioners can identify high-risk groups and pinpoint the gaps in their care.

As diversity in our population grows, the blending of these rich cultures not only will enhance the world we live in, but also create a variety of problems that need to be addressed. One of the major problems is how to communicate across cultural boundaries and create trust, particularly in the case of a life-threatening disease like cancer. To be faced with your own mortality is frightening enough, but not understanding how to participate actively in the decision making about your care is even more frightening. We should all be thankful that there are people working hard to find a solution to these problems.

This book is about life and love and hope and dreams -- the dreams of my beloved Jerry and me, being able to continue to carry the gift of survivorship and caregiving to the far corners of the United States and Canada. This certainly beats sitting on our front porch in rocking chairs talking about the "good old days."

Since Jerry and I took to the road as Speakers for Life™, we've participated in all types of media interviews. Whether the interview is for radio, television or print media, the interviewer always asks why I think I have survived all these years while so many others haven't. My standard answer is always the same: "Because no other woman will wear my jewelry." And if you know me, you know I mean every word of it.

While the challenges that survivors meet are never easy, I like to think of them as little pebbles in the path of life. I want to live and I will do everything I possibly can not only to survive, but also to enjoy life to the utmost. I may have cancer, but cancer doesn't have me and never will. I'm still looking ahead to the next bend in the road.

There's a wonderful booklet by the late Norman Vincent Peale that everyone should read, survivors and caregivers alike. It's called, "Expect a Miracle -- Make Miracles Happen." He calls this the miracle principle and he explains it this way: "If you keep your eyes open expectantly every day for great and wonderful things to happen, it is astonishing that great and wonderful things will tend to happen to you. Always think of the best. Never think of the worst. And if the worst invades your consciousness, think of it in terms of how to make it the best."

As Jerry always says, "You who are cancer survivors and caregivers have already prepared for the worst. Now go out and prepare for the best." If we all look together for that one miracle, perhaps it will be a cure for cancer.

24

Jerry's Story . . .

Prepare for the Best

Many years after her breast cancer surgery and chemotherapy, Bobbi and I were talking after dinner one night when she startled me with a question.

"Did you ever realize," she asked, "how much you hurt me when I was recovering from my surgery and I would ask you, 'Where are we going to eat Saturday night?' and you'd always put me off by saying something like, 'Well, let's wait and see,' or 'We'll talk about it later in the week,' or 'I'll think about it.'"

Ever since we were married, Bobbi and I have always eaten out on Saturday night and we still do. It's not always some place fancy but it's something we've always enjoyed doing.

So her question caught me completely by surprise. "I'm sorry," I said. "I never meant to hurt you. It was just me procrastinating as usual and never making a decision before I absolutely have to. I never meant anything by it."

"I know," she said, "but it really hurt at the time. It always seemed like you were saying, 'Let's see how she's doing later in the week,' or 'Let's see what she feels up to,' or 'Let's make sure she's still around on Saturday night.' It sounded like you were always preparing for the worst."

The statement shocked me and began to prey on my mind. Was that what I was subconsciously doing? Preparing for the worst? Why? The more I thought about it, the more a marvelous idea began to form in my head. It was so simple and so obvious and yet the more I thought about it the more I wanted to share it with others. And it all can be summed up in one short sentence. . .

"Take time right now to prepare for the -- BEST."

Everyone already knows about preparing for the worst. The whole insurance industry is built on the premise. We insure our lives, and our homes, and our cars, and our health, and our businesses, and our television sets and even our lawnmowers. And there's nothing wrong with any of that.

What I'm suggesting is that there's even more to be gained by flipping that age old adage around, and starting to prepare for the best. You who are survivors and caregivers already have faced the worst and you're reading this as living proof that there really *is* life after diagnosis Now prepare for the best. . .

    Talk about it.
      Plan it.
        Write it down.
         Do it!

When you stop and think about it, preparing for the best is better than insurance because the premium you pay is the price of enjoyment. . .the price of doing those things you always wanted to do, or wanted to do more often.

The choice is yours. Maybe it's something simple but important like spending more time with your grandchildren, or spending more time with mom and dad. Maybe it's taking that trip you've always postponed, to Alaska or Hawaii, or you name the place. Maybe it's learning to sing and joining the choir at church. . .or writing a poem or a book about your cancer experience. Maybe you've always wanted to become a nurse, or study law, or learn to fly an airplane.

It's entirely up to you. But whatever it is, do it! Start right now.

The saddest mistake of all is to do nothing. And then one day, 15 or 20 years from now, you wake up in the morning and think back over your life and exclaim, "Wow, I can't believe I made it for so long." And all you have to show for it is the scar from your surgery--and a wish list of things you always wanted to do that never got done.

You can do better than that. If you are a cancer survivor or a cancer caregiver, you're *different*. You're special. You know that cancer is *not* a death sentence. It's a wakeup call--and what you make of it is up to you, survivor and caregiver alike.

Prepare for the best--and celebrate each new day as a priceless possession because someday--someday soon, I pray--the sun is going to rise on a day when all of us-- survivors, caregivers, doctors, nurses, researchers, families and friends--will all be victors together and cancer will be nothing more than a vanishing memory of the past.

Prepare for the best!